D0814394

Getting There,
Staying There

To Pat

Getting There, Staying There

How Looking at Weight Loss Differently Changed My Life

Jennifer Klein

Enjoy!

Jennifer Klein

Thomson Publications

ISBN: 0-9709439-0-3

Library of Congress Control Number: 2001-131959

Cover: Pearl & Associates

Book design and production: Tabby House

Photo of Jennifer and dog, back cover and in montage,
© Kindra Clineff Photography

Cover photo: Peter A. Smith Photography

Acknowledgments

For his encouragement and unflinching support during the writing of this book, I will forever be grateful to my husband, Chris. His faith in me made this project possible. My mother stood by my side throughout, reminding me to be patient, assuring me that there *were* people who would accept and appreciate the information I had to share. Thanks to my friend and editor, Lisa P. Flanagan, who spent over a year reading and rereading this book. If that isn't dedication, what is? And I offer a big round of applause to Josh Criss of Precision Video, for the superior quality of his work.

And, for their generosity of spirit, I thank my clients. By bravely sharing their very personal experiences, they taught me things I could never have learned on my own. Thanks to them I now know that those of us who have struggled with our weight have countless things in common, including the ability to succeed.

Thomson Publications
5 Bedford St.
P.O. Box 706
Burlington, MA 01803

Contents

Introduction

At age eight, I was put on my first diet by our family physician. That marked the beginning of a long and painful dieting history. Like most chronic dieters, I survived on hope. Maybe the *next* diet . . . . And, because none of them worked long-term, there was *always* a next diet.

I tried every diet available and, in desperation, sometimes resorted to unsafe and gimmicky weight-loss techniques. It was a frustrating and discouraging way to live.

As an adult—in spite of years of sacrifices made in the name of weight loss—I found myself heavier than I had ever been. Overwhelmed, I finally asked myself, *What have all these years of dieting accomplished? I've lost and regained, lost and regained hundreds of pounds. Every single dieting strategy has failed. I have to be doing something* wrong. But what?

That question changed my life. I suddenly found myself in the center of a place I had never known before—a new, solidly balanced position of commitment to me. I knew I had to change my life, but for the first time that awareness made me feel powerful. I had discovered a new, rational inner voice. *Jennifer, changing your life is a process, not a race. You are capable of achieving your weight-loss goals. Sure, you'll slip at times. You'll get discouraged. There will even be days when you sabotage yourself, but none of that matters. Focus on your goal and you can still succeed.*

And I did.

This book shares the most important things I learned during my journey to weight-loss success. It explores the "make" or "break" issues, the pitfalls that affect every chronic dieter.

Because I am a weight-loss coach, I also share some of my clients' experiences as well as tips that will help prepare you—both mentally and physically—for weight loss.

Striving to reach your personal fitness goal is an adventure. It's a challenge that can actually be enjoyable, while providing countless rewards. I'm very happy that you've decided to give yourself the gift of weight loss. Congratulations.

1

Why We're Different

All or Nothing at All

I was invited to a wedding. I was worried. Social situations where food is involved always make me nervous. Very nervous. I have several "trigger foods," foods that set me off and lead to out-of-control eating. Cheese is one of them.

What if they serve cheese?

As I left for the wedding, I gave myself a strict order: *No cheese.* Cheese is my number one trigger food. I didn't dare eat it. I simply couldn't have it and that was that.

I felt in control, confident—until I saw the gigantic, golden pyramid of cheese at the buffet.

"Okay, *one* piece. Just one," I told myself.

It tasted sooooo good. I began to bargain with myself. *One more won't hurt.* Then, I promised myself, *I will stop.*

The next thing I knew I had entered the "numb zone." I was no longer in touch with myself—my body or my brain. I was spiraling out of control. One piece became five, then ten. By the time I stopped I had eaten nearly forty cubes of cheese. Forty cubes!

Would I ever have a normal relationship with food?

Here's the surprise. This episode, this feeding frenzy, this out-of-control event, took place *after* I had lost more than seventy pounds, reached my ideal weight and maintained it for *more than eight years.*

Ten years ago I weighed over two hundred pounds, though I'm only five feet two. Today, though I'm at my ideal weight, I still occasionally have out-of-control episodes with food.

Hunger Meter

Everyone is born with a "hunger meter," the name I've given the inner gauge that's *supposed* to register hunger, fullness, and everything in between. Mine is defective. It generally operates in extremes. I know "starving." I know "stuffed." I don't know genuine hunger. *I know when I should stop eating and I know when I've eaten "enough," but I don't always stop.* And, when it should, my hunger meter doesn't register "full." I often don't recognize the difference between "wanting" food and "needing" food.

I used to think this problem was unique to me. But after six years of coaching others, I learned that all of us who struggle with our weight have the same problem.

We all have a defective hunger meter.

When I started my weight-loss business I was nutrition focused. *Just show people what to eat*, I thought, *and you'll solve their weight problem. Just help people learn the difference between healthy and unhealthy food.*

But client after client told me the same thing, "I know what I *should* eat, Jennifer. I just don't know how to stop!"

When I shared my hunger meter analogy, clients were always surprised and relieved. They agreed—that defective little gauge gets us into trouble with food. I've been able to maintain my goal weight for over eight years because I've learned to compensate for my defective hunger meter.

People who are thin by nature (those annoying people who have *never* had a weight problem) have an inner gauge that works properly. Their hunger meter tells them that half a sandwich is enough to satisfy their hunger. Their gauge whispers, "Leave the rest of that food on your plate. This dinner portion is too big. If you eat all of it you'll feel uncomfortable."

I'd do anything to have that gift. That's how I see it, a gift. The ability to walk away from food. The ability to stop eating *before* I overeat, *before* I feel very uncomfortable.

My mother and I went out to eat. (She's worn a size four her entire adult life.) I ordered my favorite dinner; she ordered shrimp. I cleaned my plate, as usual. She left two shrimp on her plate, and casually pushed it aside. I stared at it. Was she finished?

"Mom, you have some shrimp left on your plate."

"Yes, I know."

"Aren't you going to finish them before the waitress takes your plate?"

"No, Jennifer. I've had enough to eat."

Now, what in the world does *that* mean? She had *enough*? Yeah, so what? There were only two little shrimp left on her plate. Why let them go to waste? I was confused. "Why don't you just finish the little bit that's left?"

"Because, I'm not hungry. Do you want them, Jennifer?"

I felt embarrassed. She had seen me finish my meal and was probably wondering why I took an interest in what she did and did not eat. She wasn't *hungry*? What does that mean? What does that feel like? She should feel "full" like me. It made no sense. When it came to eating, *full* or *stuffed* were the only words I understood.

I became defensive. "Noooo, I don't want them. I just don't see the point. Why leave two little shrimp?"

We stared at each other. We were beings from different planets. She was an alien with two heads. She wasn't "normal" and I couldn't relate to her.

But I think at that moment I also began to "get it."

I had spent much of my life complaining about the way she ate. *She eats Ben and Jerry's ice cream and she doesn't gain weight! She puts cream in her coffee, and eats chocolate! She cooks with oil and butter! She breaks every rigid weight-loss rule there is and she's never had a weight problem! I struggle to follow every diet rule, and I'm overweight!*

Why?

She knows *when* to stop. I don't.

My older brother ate like my mom—and still does. He, too, was thin—still is. He ate peanut butter sandwiches, fatty crackers, cheese, cookies, but he never gained weight. He, like my mother, breaks all the "rules." But he, like my mother, knows when to stop.

There are still times when I'm aware that I'm feeling full and heading towards stuffed (having to undo the button on my pants to breathe) but I continue to eat.

In the past I prayed, "Please, send me a miracle diet that will fix my screwed-up hunger meter." I spent thousands of dollars on diet plans hoping they would somehow give me control over food.

These expensive commercial plans did work . . . short term. The diet industry is built around the promise of control. It doesn't help us with our problem; it just focuses on our symptoms. These fad diet plans aren't designed to be a "cure." They're designed to keep us coming back over and over again. And they do, because without rigid guidelines and rules that give us *strict control* and guidance, we feel helpless. What we really need, but never get, are guidelines for life-long behavioral changes.

I know because I've been there. I was in a continuous search for the *one* diet that could change *me*, the *one* plan that would provide me with the same control my mom, brother, and other naturally lean people had. Where was the diet that would make me want to leave the two shrimp on my plate? "Oh my, I'm feeling a tad uncomfortable. I mustn't eat those two itty-bitty shrimp."

I never found that diet.

Eventually I figured out that it wasn't about control for my mom. It was natural behavior. Food, to my mother was just that—food. She ate it when she needed it.

I used to get angry with myself. Why did I eat when I wasn't hungry? Why did I snack when I was bored? What was wrong with me? Why didn't I have any willpower?

When I was off a diet, my relationship with food was frightening. It was often completely out of control.

For me, trying to figure out when and when not to eat was like driving across a desert in a car with a defective fuel gauge. Scary. Would I, did I, need fuel? Would I make it to my destination on the other side of that big, wide, open wasteland where there was no safety zone, no help, no map?

That's the reason I went back again and again to diet plans and other structured programs. They made me feel safe, in control. I was given specific food choices, told when to eat, how much to eat, and a rigid time frame for weight loss. They provided strict rules. I stayed in control because I was also held accountable. I had to climb on their scale every week. I liked having that structure because without a hunger meter I could trust, trying to diet without a plan was one big guessing game. Unfortunately, none of that structure, in the form of diets, worked.

I finally achieved my goal weight because I learned to accept the truth. My weight problem wasn't about poor willpower or failed diets. It was about my personal relationship with food and the answer to my weight problem lay in learning how to deal with it.

I've currently been at my goal size for more than eight years. Do I relate to food like a naturally lean person? No way! I doubt that I ever will. But that hasn't stopped me from maintaining my dream size.

Food still talks to me. It calls my name. It still makes me feel: feel anxious; feel happy; feel numb; feel disgusting; feel angry and feel guilty.

These are the non-hunger reasons I eat:

- I eat when I'm **bored**. Nothing to do? Let's see what's in the fridge.
- I eat when I'm **craving something**. When I have a yearning for a specific taste.
- I eat when I'm **stressed**. Frazzled after a hard day? What will comfort me? Food!
- I eat most when I'm feeling **out of control**. Stuffing myself, I end up spiraling downward until I hit rock bottom. Only then am I ready to regain control.

After working one on one with hundreds of clients I've learned that almost all of us who are overweight share these eating behaviors. We eat for many different reasons. Hunger is last on our list. For a naturally thin person it's about *needing* food not *craving* food. For them it's about "hungry or satisfied." The first reason they eat is a practical one. They have no emotional attachment to food.

New clients often say, "Jennifer, I need to work one on one with you to see if you can help me. You see, I'm different. I don't eat like a regular person. I know what I should and should not be eating. That's not my problem. My problem is I don't know when to stop."

I was amazed by the number of people who suffered the same experiences I suffered. I was very surprised to learn my out-of-balance relationship with food was more common than I ever imagined!

We Know

- *Overweight people know* fast food at midnight isn't a formula for weight loss.
- *Overweight people know* that eating one piece of pizza is better than eating four.
- *Overweight people know* that adding butter and sour cream to a baked potato makes it higher in fat and calories than a plain potato.
- *Overweight people know* that fatty salad dressing should be ordered on the side and used sparingly.
- *Overweight people know* that one serving of food is better than two or three.
- *Overweight people know* at least as much about basic nutrition as thin people.

The clients I coach have a common problem. They're trying to lose weight and keep it off. They're struggling with the same eating behaviors I have. It's not just about what we eat; it's about *how much* we eat and our *reasons* for eating. We share the same *eating behaviors*, triggered by different things, but they all result in an out-of-control relationship with food.

There is no diet that will fix our defective hunger meter. Learning to live with that reality is part of the solution. There *is* a way for us to lose weight and maintain weight loss—despite our inability to recognize when we need food and when we want food.

This book will help you cope with your out-of-balance food relationship. It will teach you to think differently. You will learn to evaluate true weight-loss success. It will guide you in eliminating destructive habits and help you to develop structure in your eating patterns.

"They" Don't Understand

A doctor and I were having a discussion about diet pills. I said, "I think it's wrong for doctors to prescribe weight-loss pills. Overweight people are going to be dealing with food issues for the rest of their lives. Diet pills just provide a quick fix."

I knew he prescribed diet drugs and I wanted him to know this disappointed me. His unsympathetic answer confirmed my suspicion: naturally thin people can't relate to what we go through.

"What am I supposed to do with these people, Jennifer?" he asked. "Sometimes I want to yell, 'Stop eating so much!' But they don't listen when I suggest they eat less. Pills will do the work I can't!"

He was lean and fit, had never had a weight problem, and he didn't know I had taken off more than seventy pounds. I was offended by his comments at first, but then I realized that someone who has never had a weight problem couldn't understand what it's like to struggle with weight. To him, we were people who just couldn't get enough food. Why couldn't we just stop eating too much? He actually believed it was that simple.

And he's not alone in his opinion. Many people are confused when I describe my business. "You counsel and coach people for weight loss? You talk to people about food?" They give the same response my doctor friend did. "Why don't you just tell them to stop eating so much?"

We already know we need to eat less, don't we?

Most of the people who sell us weight-loss advice—including the impractical, unrealistic, or unsafe kind—have never had a weight problem. In spite of that, we take their advice because we assume they have the answer.

Wrong!

If you've never "been there" you don't know what overeating is *really* about. The doctor at the gym assumed, as many people do, that we don't know what to eat, don't know how to cut fat, and haven't figured out that we must exercise.

But, the fact is, we already know all that!

Everyone reading this book knows what to do. At my peak weight I did. I knew that polishing off a box of cookies wasn't going to get me into the size of my dreams. I knew that cleaning my plate when I was already stuffed was not a formula for weight loss. So, why did I do it?

But I Could Learn

After I had gone away to school, I returned home for a visit and discovered a pint of New York Super Fudge Chunk ice cream in my mom's freezer. I was trying to change my eating habits. It took tremendous willpower, but I managed to shut the freezer door. I didn't want to attack the pint. The ice cream was on my mind during the whole visit. It called to me, but I made it through the visit without a bite! I was so proud!

About three months later I went home again. I opened the freezer and saw another pint of New York Super Fudge Chunk. Whoa! Had Mom developed some food issues of her own? (I hate to admit it, but I would have been secretly pleased—misery loves company.)

"Wow, Mom," I said, "You're really liking that ice cream, huh?"

"Oh, I forgot it was in there."

I stood in silence, my mouth hanging open.

Yes, it was the *same* pint from three months earlier. Obviously she's insane! The fact is, naturally thin people have no emotional attachment to food. I can't say it often enough. The availability of the ice cream meant nothing. She had forgotten all about it.

I wouldn't have forgotten. That pint of ice cream would have haunted me daily until it was gone.

Jennnnnn. Jennnnn. Come finish me, Jennnnn. Eat me aaall uuuup!

I would have thought about that ice cream constantly, eventually yanking the container from the freezer and finishing it once and for all. To my mother it was nothing but ice cream: a paper carton with stuff inside. That's it. No haunting voices, no guilt attached to taking a bite, just ice cream.

What's your seductive food? Could you forget about ice cream? I might—if it was tuna flavored!

Gradually, I became aware that naturally thin people, people without food issues, didn't have the emotional attachment to food I had.

While in college, I worked in the restaurant business. I got to know a chef, a very *thin* chef. Often we'd take our break together. He ate the same snack, the same way, every day.

He'd saunter up to the vending machine. He'd reach into his pocket and pull out some change. After feeding the coins into the machine, he'd press the button for peanut butter cups. He'd wait for the candy to fall, casually pick it up, then walk back to the table and place the candy bar in front of him. He'd talk with us co-workers for a while. Then, after about five minutes, he would slowly open the candy bar.

He'd break one of the peanut butter cups into fours. "Anybody want a piece?" he'd ask. Most of the time people said, "No thanks."

I'd be thinking, *No, I don't want a piece, I want the* whole thing. *I want everyone to disappear so I can shove the whole candy bar in my mouth.*

In about twenty minutes he'd finish *half* of the candy bar. Yes, one-half! He'd fold up the wrapper with the other half still inside and put it in his pocket. I chalked it up as another example of a "crazy" thin person in action. Who knows if he actually ate the other half! Maybe he'd forget it was in his pocket and it would end up in the wash. Maybe he'd give the other half away. Maybe he'd throw it away. The candy bar wasn't important to him. No guilt, no emotional attachment, it was just a candy bar.

Me? I would have yanked out my change, and—feeling obliged to justify my behavior—I would have announced loudly, "PMS-ing, everyone! Gotta have my chocolate." I would have waited impatiently for the candy to hit the bottom, ripped the package open as soon as I got it in my hand, popped half in my mouth *before* I sat down (offering it to no one—or if I did, the offer was phony) and devour the other half in a matter of seconds.

Then I'd feel guilty. *I blew it! How could I be so stupid? Candy's not on my diet!* Self-destruction would begin. *Well, I already ate one candy bar, I might as well have one more.* But I wouldn't stop there.

After stuffing myself with candy, my judgmental, negative voice would shout, *I can't believe you did that, Jennifer! You know you shouldn't have had all that candy.* The resulting anger, self-disgust, and frustration would send me into an emotional downward spiral. It wasn't until I felt thoroughly defeated that I could begin to dig myself out of my pit of self-loathing and prepare to start being "perfect" with food once again.

Unlike the chef, for me it wasn't just about candy, it was also about a "rebellious" decision. It was about indulging myself in a way that wasn't good for me. Abandoning control. Giving in. It was about being "bad." I sincerely believed that *not* eating the candy was "good"; eating the candy was "bad." There were no choices in between.

You know how it goes. Once we make the decision to "give up" and "give in" there's no stopping us.

Fear of Starvation

To celebrate something—I can't remember exactly what—my parents took me to a very fancy and expensive French restaurant. *Wow, this is gonna be good*, I thought. When the waiter brought my entree, I stared at it in disbelief. There on a large white plate, was the smallest bite of salmon I'd ever seen. Next to it lay a teaspoon of spinach and a tiny dollop of potatoes. *What's this?* I felt cheated. I began to panic. I would starve! Why bother to eat this meal? I frantically began to plan a *real* meal I could eat when I got home.

For those of us with portion issues, this reaction is common. My clients have shown me that fear of not getting enough is an emotion that many overweight people share. We like to see quantity. If we don't see a lot of food on our plate we assume we won't be satisfied. When we see a small portion, we feel deprived even before we take that first bite.

Seventy pounds ago, I had the opportunity to vacation in Holland. While sight-seeing, friends and I went to lunch. I ordered a sandwich. When the waitress brought it, I went into shock. What had they brought me? There on my plate sat a piece of bread the size of a small dinner roll. On it lay one little piece of meat, and one tiny slice of cheese. "They call this a sandwich?"

No one else at my table seemed to notice how small their serving was. No one else was obsessed about food. No one else on the trip had a weight problem. Everyone else was enjoying the scenery and the company.

I can trace my "fear of not getting enough" back to age six.

In the grade school cafeteria, the sign over the bread bin read LIMIT 6. The pieces of bread were small, and I would grab the allowed six slices at once. Then I would turn to the kid next to me. If he or she hadn't taken their share of slices, I would ask for them. I have vivid memories of these behaviors. My eating was frantic. I always wanted more than "enough." I always wanted big amounts of everything . . . except fruits and vegetables.

Another vivid memory illustrates this fear. My mother had cooked hot dogs and baked beans. She and my father were going out for the evening, leaving my brother and me with a baby-sitter. I was about eight.

The sitter served our dinner. I finished mine quickly and went to the stove for a second helping. As I was walking back to the table the sitter stopped me. She knelt in front of me and placed her hands on my shoulders. I felt nervous. What was she doing?

"Jennifer, don't eat that second plate of food. Look at me. Do you want to end up like me?" She was an overweight and unhappy teenager. She wanted to spare me the struggles she'd had.

I remember moving out of her way to get to the table. I was carrying my second helping and I was determined to eat it. This was the first time my weight problem had taken a "direct hit" from someone other than kids at school or my brother. I was hurt and shocked. I wanted her to leave me alone.

That event has stuck with me for twenty-five years. Remembering it makes me feel sad. She was trying to help me before my weight problem got worse. But her thoughtfulness and concern had made me uncomfortable. Instead of making me want to change my behaviors, her advice had made me defensive and angry. I was fully aware of my weight problem. Other kids reminded me of it, in a mean way, every day. But *I* was the only one who was allowed to say anything to *me* about my weight. It was too private and delicate an issue to discuss with anyone else. Besides, I was a long way from being ready to deal with it.

Today I remember that baby-sitter as an overweight person who made a kind gesture. She was convinced, based on her own experience, that if my eating behaviors continued, I would forever be struggling with my weight.

Unfortunately, weight problems in childhood appear more and more common. As an adult, I've seen my early, unbalanced eating behaviors in many children.

Recently, at a party, I noticed a very chubby little girl. She was about five years old, already about twenty pounds overweight. She was dressed like a little princess, a mass of curly blonde hair gathered, in a beautiful pink bow, at the top of her head.

I was in the buffet line when she wedged her body between me and the person ahead of me. She took pepperoni, piece after piece, until her plate was piled high. I stepped back and watched her. She was eating just like me as a child; she was me in the grade school cafeteria line, taking as much bread as I could get. The look on her face said the pepperoni meant the world to her.

When do unhealthy relationships with food begin? This little girl's mother was also overweight. Did she share her mother's food behaviors? Nature versus nurture? What was my excuse? Remember my mom, the woman with the two shrimp left on her plate? I was never encouraged to eat *anything* I didn't want.

What if there is no universal answer? The reasons may be different for each of us, but the behaviors are the same.

I have clients who were overweight as children. I have clients who were thin until they had children of their own. I have other clients whose unhealthy eating habits started in college. Still others who didn't start gaining weight until later in life.

For some people the hunger meter breaks early in life. For others, it slowly starts to break down over time. And for people who eat only what they need, those people who have never had a weight problem, it operates just fine. Lucky them!

It's Always with You

Once I finally succeeded at "getting there and staying there," I didn't suddenly exclaim, "My God, I've got it! I know hunger! I know what it means to be satisfied! I know when to stop eating! My hunger meter works! Food has no emotional hold on me! A pint of ice cream no longer calls to me! I can forget it's there! I can leave shrimp on my plate! My problems are over!"

WRONG!

Though my emotional attachment to food did change over time, my defective hunger meter relationship with food has *never* gone away. But I have learned to work with it. Take it from me, an inability to distinguish genuine hunger doesn't have to stop you from staying at your ideal size.

You can develop new, healthier ways to deal with food. That's what I learned to do. And that's why I was able to lose weight and keep it off, and help others who have struggled with weight do the same thing.

No matter how discouraged, frustrated, and hopeless you feel, remember I've been where you are. I gave up and started again countless times before I finally achieved lasting success. I've followed the plans, done the diets, popped the pills. Often frustrated, I asked myself, "Is losing weight worth it?"

It is.

If you repeatedly approach weight loss as a battle or a struggle you'll be fighting with your self-destructive behaviors for the rest of your life. Think of weight loss as a challenge, a learning experience. Let go of the win-the-war mentality. The mind change comes first. Weight loss will follow.

You Can Succeed

I am proof that a very overweight person can learn to find *balance* and *control* in a healthy, permanent way.

Yes, it's *me* saying this, the girl who visited the local convenient mart with a fake list of names, a fictional list of people who had *supposedly* sent me to buy candy bars. I'd approach the counter, look at the clerk, hold up the list and with a straight face say, "Jimmy wants a Butterfinger, Sally wants M&Ms, Lisa wants an Almond Joy. . . ." (As if the guy behind the counter really gave a damn!) But I'd sooner have died than let him know I intended to eat every candy bar myself.

Some of my clients share similar stories: a trip through the drive-thru window with a fake list of people to explain the larger-than-normal food order or the client who always added two sodas to her double fast-food order, so the person waiting on her would think the meal was for two.

Stories like these are common. Fake lists, bogus orders, eat it all or none at all, PMS announcements, or "closet eating." These are some of the outlandish ways we deal with the guilt we attach to "bad" food behaviors.

As a teenager, my brother used to be proud when he occasionally devoured huge amounts of food. He never had—still doesn't have—any food-related guilt. Imagine any one of us with weight issues bragging about chowing down a huge amount of anything!

We're not proud of our eating habits. We know those behaviors produce weight gain. We also know what it takes to lose weight. Then why don't we lose weight and keep it off? Because deep down we are resigned to the truth: those radical methods we use to lose weight quickly were never intended to be used for a lifetime. We can pop diet pills for awhile, drink diet shakes for a few weeks, eliminate forbidden foods for as long as we can endure it, follow the fad diet plans, but eventually we will return to our old food behaviors. Since we can't live on a diet for the rest of our life, and we're not given any other options, what choice do we have?

The only *logical alternative* is to develop healthy, lifetime habits that will change the way we deal with food. Do this and the battle becomes a manageable "challenge." Food stops being the "enemy." We *will* be able to lose weight and keep it off.

2

Desperate for Control

Wait till Monday

On which day do we typically start a diet? Answer: Monday. Why Monday? Because it allows us that "last weekend" to stuff ourselves with the foods we love! We eat everything, and as much of it as we want. Why not? After all, suffering on a new diet is right around the corner.

Are you familiar with the last weekend free-for-all? "I won't be ordering foods like pizza for awhile, so why not have six slices? This is the last weekend of freedom! What about those cookies? Might as well eat three . . . six . . . eight. I'll eat them until I'm stuffed because I won't be tasting cookies for quite some time. Diet-Monday is just a weekend away.

Each time I prepared to start a diet, I'd behave like a person on a mission. I'd dedicate myself to eating all my food favorites. No limits, no restrictions. I wanted to self-destruct; I wanted to pack it *all* in while I still could. Stuff myself! I'd eat the foods I craved until I couldn't taste them anymore. My goal was to be as bad as possible *before* I had to be absolutely perfect.

I once bought a half gallon of mint chocolate chip ice cream and a container of chocolate syrup and pigged-out, eating it straight from the carton! Chocolate syrup dribbled down my chin. I was like a two-year-old having her first ice cream experience. Pizza? I'd eat it. Regular soda? I'd gulp it. I'd stuff myself with chips, candy, all kinds of junk. I'd shock myself with the amount I could eat! Sometimes, I'd end up sick. When breathing became a challenge, I'd have to change my clothes for comfort's sake. Loose elastic was always my fashion choice.

It was easy to rationalize my bad pre-diet behavior. I knew I wouldn't be allowed to eat *any* of my favorite delicious, satisfying foods for several weeks, maybe *months*! "Jennifer," I'd tell myself, "you deserve these treats. You'll have to be in complete control starting Monday."

I'd spend those pre-diet weekends eating *so much*, and feeling *so bad* that I would actually begin to look forward to my diet. I was eager to start feeling comfortable again, healthier and better about myself. The final surrender of my rebellious eating behaviors to a diet was always a part of my weight-loss game.

After years of coaching other chronic dieters, I've learned I'm also not alone in these behaviors. One client called these behaviors, "The last weekend of fun." "The Last Supper," another joked. "Eat it all, 'cause soon it will be none at all!" is a common pre-diet philosophy.

When I introduce a new client to my approach to weight loss, I explain that before we design a *realistic* food plan that fits their lifestyle, I need to see a list of what they typically eat in a week. I ask them to write down what they eat when they're *not* preparing to start a diet—a normal week. "Pretend we haven't met," I tell them. "Just be yourself."

I always ask about the nature of their day, because it's important.

- Is it hectic?
- Do they let themselves get excessively hungry?
- How much cooking do they do?
- When do they eat?
- What types of foods do they typically choose?
- What are their favorite foods?
- How often do they eat out?
- When do they eat the most?

I look for patterns of behavior. Getting an honest record of what my clients normally eat can be very difficult. Many of them have a pre-diet mind-set. "I'm working with Jennifer so I'm going to be told that I can't have certain foods after this week. I'd better eat this now, for the *last* time."

They find it difficult to abandon that I'm-about-to-suffer mentality. We dieters always assume the worst. I call it the prepare-to-starve mind-set.

One new client, "Mary," provided me with her food-tracking information. Her sheet looked like a menu from a fast-food restaurant.

"Mary," I asked, "do you typically eat fast food four nights a week?"

"Well, no, but I figured I'd have one last fling before I started my diet! I'm not really *that* bad, I just wanted to eat burgers and fries, pizza, and other good stuff for one last time."

"Josephine" spent her food-chart week melting cheese on *everything*! She melted it on bread, pasta, vegetables, and even pretzels. I asked, "Is this dedication to cheese-melting typical behavior?"

"No, but I wanted to finish the four bags of shredded cheese that were in the refrigerator. I didn't want them to go to waste."

"Patty" was on the chocolate chip cookie plan. According to her food-tracking sheets, Patty had cookies for breakfast, lunch, dinner, and late evening snacks. Did she normally average between six to ten cookies a day?

"I rarely eat them," she insisted. "But because they're my absolute favorite, I spent hours baking with my kids." She ate nearly three-dozen cookies on her own! She was sure that no weight-loss plan was going to allow her to eat chocolate chip cookies.

Not everyone self-destructs to this degree, but self-destructive food behaviors seem to be part of our nature. I'll bet you've had the "splurge before Monday" pre-diet experience. We prepare to suffer. We begin a weight-loss plan the way a soldier prepares for battle—having that last hurrah while fearing the worst.

Is it any wonder why we dieters want to finish a diet as soon as possible? We can't bear to be without our favorite foods for long. We're not prepared to suffer forever. In other words, we're *normal*. Why would *anyone* agree to suffer indefinitely, unless there was something wrong with them? Why should we *suffer* at all? That's a very important question. The truth is that healthy, lean people don't "suffer" in order to stay the way they are. Remember my mother, the thin person? If she wants a cookie, she *eats* a cookie. She makes no judgments about it. It's just a cookie. The thing that's absent for her is the good/bad judgment call. She doesn't evaluate food as she eats it. She doesn't eat something she wants and then beat herself up. She doesn't try to control her food intake. Even if she does eat a lot of something, she doesn't declare herself "out of control." Control isn't an issue. Food (and getting control of it) isn't the focus of her life. For us, food has all the power.

Occasionally we perpetual dieters pin our food behaviors down, for awhile. But, because we're so rigid when we're "in control," we require ourselves to be perfect. That doesn't work because it's too hard! Who can live in a constant state of perfection? It's impossible to stay in *perfect* control.

It's also completely unrealistic.

When I finally began my successful weight loss, I chose to approach it differently than I had in the past. My first positive step? I decided to begin this new weight-loss plan midweek. I knew I had to eliminate that "dramatic" Monday start. I began my seventy-pound weight loss on a Thursday.

One by one, I was going to examine every dieting technique that had failed me in the past. I would try to figure out where the flaws were and correct them. Starting my weight loss on a Thursday instead of a Monday was one small change that was part of my major change in strategy.

We Have a Wait Problem!

Every time I started a new diet—and, believe me, I started *hundreds* of them—I was prepared to suffer and resigned to be miserable.

With an average of seventy pounds to lose, I usually approached a diet determined to reach my weight-loss goal within five to six months. As long as I was convinced I could reach my goal *fast,* I could face beginning another new struggle.

I hated being on a diet, but without the structure a diet provided I had no willpower. When I managed to find some willpower it wouldn't last long. I'd always return to my old bad habits. That's why, if a diet promised quick results, I repeatedly signed up without hesitation. It didn't matter what I was advised to eat, to drink, to mix, to combine, to avoid, or to measure. My focus was always the same: *fast results.* How long would I have to stay on the diet to reach my weight-loss goal?

And my game plan never changed. I always stuffed myself just before starting a diet. Then once I was on the diet, I was frantic to take the weight off as quickly as possible, because part of me was always terrified that I would fail.

I've learned, through my clients, that self-doubt plagues most dieters. We commit to a diet wondering how long we'll be able to stick with it. I couldn't stick to any of them for long. Generally I'd stay on a diet about one to two months before calling it quits. After abandoning the diet with nowhere else to go, I'd return to my out-of-control food behaviors.

The pressure was always on to lose as much weight as I could before returning to my old familiar ways. Personally, I wanted a fast way out of the body I had come to hate.

The diet industry hooks us with promises of "fast": "Lose 30 pounds in **30 days!**" "Lose all the weight you want in just **six weeks!**" "Sleep off the pounds **overnight!**"

I was a sucker for gimmicks, especially ones that promised speedy results. I signed up for every one! *Fast* and *easy* was the light at the end of my dreaded weight-loss tunnel. "Fast" made me optimistic about starting a diet. I could see the finish line. "This diet is unbearable, but I *am* losing lots of weight. Thank God I won't be on it for long!" Accept the truth: *fast does not last.*

When we begin a diet, we're not thinking about the rest of our lives. When we're on a diet, we think only about the *diet.* We focus on the foods we're supposed to eat and the ones we're not supposed to eat. We're dependent on the structure, the restrictions, and the rules we've been told to follow.

There's a lot of "busy work" involved in most diets. The busy work makes the process feel exciting and challenging. We convince ourselves that, for that short period of diet-time, we are *really* accomplishing something. It's a false sense of accomplishment. Some statistics suggest that more than 90 percent of dieters regain all weight lost within one year! What does that tell us? Unless we focus on changing our *behaviors*, we'll be dieting over and over again . . . forever!

Like most dieters, I always set a *specific* weight-loss goal with a plan to reach it in a *specific* amount of time. "Okay, Jennifer," I'd tell myself, "you should be down *at least* twenty pounds by the end of next month! And by the time summer arrives, you should have reached your weight-loss goal!"

I was the queen of high-pressure/time-limit, weight loss. When I made the decision to lose weight, a frantic person took control. In my mind I would hear her screaming, *Get the weight off now! I hate this body and I don't want to look at it for one more day!*

I didn't know about the frantic nature of the overweight until I started working one on one with my clients. We chronic dieters want our weight to come off fast. We want it off easy, and we want it off yesterday.

By making *time* our focus, we often destroy all our hard work. Our negative voices say, *It's been three months, why do I look the same? Why! The last time I tried to lose weight I was down fifteen pounds in two months! This time I'm only down ten pounds! I'm trying so hard, and this weight loss is going so slowly. I might as well just QUIT!*

Changing your body requires working slowly to correct *years* of unhealthy habits. You're being unrealistic and unfair to yourself if you believe a lifetime of bad habits can be changed in a few days, weeks, or even months.

I measure my clients on a monthly basis. "Lisa" was losing weight very slowly. On average she lost an inch a month in her most difficult area—her hips. I assumed, like most of my clients, Lisa needed a pep talk because her weight loss was going slowly. Part of my job is keeping clients from becoming discouraged. "Lisa," I said, "don't worry, you're still heading in the right direction."

Her positive answer surprised me. "Hey, I figure if I only lose one inch a month, in fifteen months I'll have thirty-six-inch hips! I'll look as good as I did in college!" With her positive and patient attitude, I knew Lisa would make it to her goal.

As I explained, my first session with clients is called "Getting to Know You." During this session we discuss the clients' weight, diet, and health history. We discuss their food and exercise habits. Do they exercise? What activities do they enjoy? Have they always struggled with their weight? What's their family's weight history? When do they eat? What are their favorite foods?

I don't offer a new client any guidance or advice relating to food, until the *second week* on the program. I have them track an average food week *before* we start to change old habits. When I explain that this is my policy, new clients almost always panic.

"Jennifer! You want me to eat what I've been eating for another whole week?! I thought you'd put me on a diet today! I have to get started as soon as possible! I've been out of control!"

When we are at the lowest of low in self-esteem and self-control, we want a plan that gives us instant results. We want an immediate turnaround. We want strict control.

At this point we're ready and willing to set goals for ourselves that are not just unrealistic, they're cruel.

Imagine hearing someone say, "You are going to learn to ski with the *experts*. For three months you'll have the use of a tow rope. Grab it and hold on."

Holding onto the tow rope gets you up and down the slopes. You feel as if you are skiing like the experts and the method is fast and easy!

After three weeks you're comfortable on the slopes. You perform well as long as you use the "towrope."

But now the three months are up. You have to let go of the rope. Suddenly you realize you haven't learned anything. You've just been pulled where you wanted to go. You have no skills. But you're supposed to head down that mountain as usual. You're terrified. Why wouldn't you be?

You're stranded at the top of the mountain. You push yourself forward. Suddenly you're in a free-fall, rolling out of control down a mountain you never had the skills to conquer.

This story demonstrates the difference between learning new eating habits and dieting.

Diet-focused clients remind me of the "old" me. They're not thinking about developing a strategy for lifelong success. They have no patience, no self-confidence, and no long-term plan. Taking the time to learn new skills is not their focus. *Just hand me that towrope* is what they're thinking.

I usually have to remind them that during our "sign-up" consultation, I explained my weight-loss philosophy. "Successful weight loss is about changing your life, learning new skills, developing new and healthier habits. It's about changing who you are, *permanently.*" If they seem worried about time, I ask them if they're really ready to make this commitment.

If they're still searching for the miracle diet, the diet that promises instant results in little time with no effort, then I ask them to examine their diet history. Where has dieting taken them? How successful were they, long-term? If they lost weight on diets in the past, how did they feel when the diet ended? Were they confident around food? What had they learned that would help them manage their food issues? If their past "fast and easy" dieting methods worked, why have they now come to me?

I understand how they feel. I often allowed "slow" results to make me quit. It was backward thinking. I'd quit because my progress was slow, then return to my old ways, usually regaining more weight than I'd lost. In a year or two, I'd start another diet.

Ironically, I never panicked about doing nothing for one to two years at a time before starting the next diet. Time was only an issue when I was preparing for a diet or actually *on* the diet. It wasn't an issue when I was eating what I wanted and gaining weight! During those "lost" two years, I could have been losing weight "slow and steady."

When I was in school I hated math, especially algebra. But I had a teacher who taught me the importance of giving myself time. She said, "Jennifer, be patient and relax. Eventually you'll begin to understand algebra. It won't intimidate you anymore."

If that same teacher had said, "Jennifer, you'd better 'get' algebra before this semester is over, or else!" I would have been frantic.

Her patient approach provided time to learn. The get-it-or-else approach would have made it unlikely that I could ever succeed.

When I explain "weight-loss time" to my clients, I use the plant analogy. I point to a beautiful ivy I have in my office. It's a lush, thick green plant.

When I first purchased the plant, it had a few tiny sprouts and very few leaves. For some reason, I bonded with this plant. It looked like it was struggling. I wanted to take care of it. I had been looking for a beautiful ivy, but this ivy needed help. I couldn't resist the urge to help it grow. I took it to my office.

I cared for it. I watered it. I opened my office shades to provide more light. I pruned its dead leaves.

I didn't evaluate its progress on a daily basis. I didn't inspect it to make sure it was growing. I just did what I knew needed to be done.

About a year later, as I prepared to water it I suddenly realized it had become beautiful.

It's likely I would have become discouraged by its slow progress if I had evaluated its growth on a daily basis. It would have seemed as though nothing was happening. But I just kept doing what it takes to care for a plant and it thrived.

Let's pretend that I approached this plant the way many people approach weight loss.

I see the plant. It looks pretty bad to me, but I decide to whip it into shape. I put it on a strict plant food diet. Only one small drop of plant food every two days. Lots of water. Lots of light. Let's get this plant where it should be.

Every day I examine the plant for new growth. There *must* be new growth. How come I don't see it?

I move the plant to a brighter window. Still no growth! Granted, there's a tiny new sprout, but that's not enough. I want to see progress! I want a new, beautiful plant *now*! Look at the effort I've gone to! Maybe I'll give the plant more water.

After another cup of water I check the plant again. The sprout is no bigger than it was yesterday! This is ridiculous. I'm really working hard on this plant and I have nothing to show for it! A whole week has gone by. It should be beautiful by now. Where are the lush new leaves? Where's the growth? All this care stuff isn't working. That's it. I'm done. The next stop for this hopeless plant is the trash.

This kind of compulsive evaluation frustrates and discourages dieters. I learned that if I ate in a balanced, healthy way, I would reach my goal and stay there—**and stay there**! I can't repeat this often enough. "Staying there" is the only *true* successful weight loss.

When I quit smoking, I phoned my mother. "Mom! It's been three weeks and two days that I haven't smoked!" What she said made me mad: "Jennifer, I'll know that you've really quit for good when you stop counting the days."

Why had she said *that*? Here I was busting my butt, avoiding people who smoked, finding other things to do with my time, agonizing over every smokeless minute and she didn't believe I was serious?

The *nerve,* I thought.

Her statement was maddening because she was right. I was still obsessing, still focused on cigarettes. Panicking. Scared that if I got my hands on a cigarette, I'd break down and smoke a pack. And it wouldn't end there. I might have another pack the next day, and smoke my brains out the day after that, until I was ready to start again. I'd lose control.

Give yourself permission to learn about yourself as you approach weight loss. Don't beat yourself up for making mistakes. Patience is your most valuable weight-loss tool.

By the way, I now have no idea when I last had a cigarette.

When I began my final weight loss I knew, realistically, it would be at least two years before I became the person I wanted to be, with the body I wanted to have. For the first time in my diet history, I wasn't approaching weight loss as a race. I had been very overweight for more than twenty years. I figured taking two years to undo twenty years of out-of-control food behavior was realistic.

Jennifer, I told myself, you can change your life. I will agree to trust "you," but you have to agree to give "me" time.

Time isn't an enemy. Give yourself the opportunity to learn from your mistakes. If you do, you can change old behaviors. You can become a new "you." You can make that familiar weight-loss pressure vanish! Weight loss can be an exciting, new experience.

Let go of being in a rush. Let go of your fears and self-doubt. You *can* reach your goal.

Poster Girl for Failure

My personal diet history isn't pretty.

I was either on a diet or off a diet all my overweight life. With over seventy pounds to lose, I was always miserable, uncomfortable, and unsure of myself. I assumed that a diet would give me the self-discipline I longed for. Some diets did that, but never for very long.

I always finished a diet looking better but feeling worse. I was never confident with my new body. I knew, deep down, I couldn't maintain the diet lifestyle.

During one failed commercial diet, I had lost thirty pounds in less than a month. The staff at the diet company actually applauded me during one of my weigh-in sessions because I had lost ten pounds in *one week*! At that point I was almost a month ahead of my goal weight-loss schedule. I was a diet superstar.

I was thrilled because I was preparing to go on vacation. Being ahead of schedule gave me a certain amount of freedom. While on vacation, I didn't have to be perfect.

I wasn't due to check in with the weight-loss staff for three weeks. Yippee! That gave me a week to undo any damage done during my vacation. And I planned to *vacation*: dinners out, drinks by the pool, hearty breakfasts, and late night buffets! I was convinced I could get away with all these things. After all, I was a superstar.

Can you guess what happened? I'll bet you can. The minute I de-planed I was like an animal released from a cage. I remember ordering a piña colada before I left the airport. I was on a mission. I was going to have a good time. Bye-bye diet. I'll be back in two weeks!

For the next two weeks, I lived in diet denial. I ate what I wanted, when I wanted and how much I wanted. Hadn't I earned it? Sure, my clothes were getting tighter, I felt heavier, but I didn't want to think about that. I pushed it to the back of my mind. Besides, I had that extra week for damage repair.

When my eat whatever/whenever vacation ended, it was a lot harder to buckle down than I thought it would be. Suddenly, I had only *four days* before I faced the weight-loss staff and the scale. Panic set in. I knew I had done *some* damage, but how much? I really didn't want to know. They had given me the label "fastest loser." The last thing I wanted was the label "fastest gainer." Now I was in a race against time.

Suddenly, *their* program wasn't radical enough. I didn't trust it to repair the damage I had done. I needed something stricter. I was prepared to punish myself for my diet-destroying behaviors. For the next four days I ate only fruit and drank only water. On the last day before "weigh-in" I ate absolutely nothing and prayed for a miracle.

It didn't work. I had gained seven pounds. I was no longer the "superstar." I hated myself. My enthusiasm was gone. I had lost all my momentum. I was demoralized.

The staff tried to pump me up. "You can lose it, Jennifer! Don't worry, one week on our plan will take care of this!"

At that point, one more week sounded like forever. I had no will left. I was defeated. All I wanted now was diet "down time." I wanted to get as far away from dieting as I could. I needed time to recover. I needed time to deal with my self-disgust.

Nearly two years passed before I was ready to attempt weight loss again.

The next time I was only willing to put in a minimal amount of effort. Commercials for liquid shake diets made success look *easy*. Busy day? No problem. I could carry cans of that stuff around with me. This program would be worry-free; there were no questions about what I could eat. What could be more convenient and simple? I was only required to eat "real food" once a day. This was the effortless diet I longed for. Open the can and drink your meal. This would be a cinch.

In no time, I lost twenty-eight pounds! I was thrilled. This diet method seemed too good to be true.

It was.

As I remember, I enjoyed my twenty-eight-pound weight loss for less than two weeks. The shakes had kept me in control, but I abandoned that diet because I couldn't stand the thought of drinking one more sip! None of my destructive food behaviors had changed and as a result, my downfall came quickly.

A friend who always stocks junky snacks invited me to visit. She offered potato chips. I hadn't had a junky snack for months. It was like tasting potato chips for the first time. What a flavor! I ate the whole bag. What else did she have to eat? Oh no, the return of the old out-of-control me! I was now on a self-destruct mission.

As the weeks passed, I gave in to every temptation. I stuffed myself with favorite foods I had been denied for months. It's that I-just-don't-care-anymore feeling every frustrated dieter has experienced. Before I knew it, I'd regained the twenty-eight pounds I'd lost.

Welcome to the lowest of lows—that place every chronic dieter knows. I was in shock. I had no faith left in myself. I *had* taken control. I *had* lost weight. I was a *successful* dieter. *How did I end up here?*

Another year passed. I was ready to try something brand-new. This time I had found the answer: a diet program that supplied the food. What a concept! Talk about control. Food was handed to me, on a weekly basis, in a plastic bag. No shopping, no cooking, just heat and *eat*! This diet plan provided everything from salad dressings to harmless desserts. All the work was done. I didn't even have to think about it!

I stayed on that special diet plan for over six months. It was very expensive, but worth it because in that time I lost an impressive fifty-five pounds! For the first time in my life I was close to my "ideal" weight.

People complimented me. They told me I looked fantastic. But, instead of enjoying their compliments, I felt terrified. And though I didn't understand *why*, I had every reason to be. I was off the diet. I had returned to eating normal food. But—once again—none of my eating *behaviors* had changed. The diet hadn't cured my unhealthy relationship with food. It wasn't designed to. Diets are designed to provide *temporary* escape from out-of-control eating habits. And that's just what they do. And the part of me that was terrified knew that.

For several months I had eaten only the food the diet program provided and had pretty much avoided social situations. On the rare occasions when I *did* socialize, I ate a *safe*, diet-plan meal before I confronted the normal food. I desperately wanted to maintain control of my eating, but I also wanted to be normal again. So, when the invitation came, I eagerly accepted a dinner date for pizza with friends. I was nervous, but I felt I could handle the pressure. I convinced myself I could limit myself to only a slice or two.

When I tasted the pizza, it was nirvana. "I'll be 'perfect' tomorrow," I promised myself, as I continued to stuff pizza into my mouth. "But today I'm going to eat what and how much I want."

Once again I was going from completely "in control" to completely "out of control." Within a week, I had regained five pounds. Then, I hit the ten-pound mark. I told myself I'd stop at ten, then I hit twenty. Thirty. I'd stop at thirty. Forty? Fifty?

My God! I weigh more now than I did when I started the diet!

I regained fifty-plus pounds in less than one year. All my hard work, gone. All the diet program money had been spent for nothing. How could I have failed—again?

Welcome back to the lowest of lows. *How did I end up here?*

After that major failure, during the following three years, I tried "magazine" diets, "soup" diets, "over-the-counter" diet pills—you name it! But none of them provided the control I was looking for. Can you believe it? . . . I was ready to go back to the food-provided diet plan. It had worked for me. It had given me total control. I was in denial. I was willing to forget about the dependency it created which made long-term, genuine success impossible.

So, I signed up for the food-provided diet plan a second time. But I wasn't able to muster the enthusiasm I'd had before. I purchased the food—now even more expensive—and started again. The plan didn't give me the exhilarating, confident feeling it had the first time. Because I had failed to maintain my weight loss, this time the promise of control sounded false, the feeling of hope was gone. I lost ten or so pounds and called it quits. Now I didn't know where to turn.

At this point, I weighed more than ever. Despite the fact that I had spent thousands of dollars on strict diet plans, I had achieved nothing.

When I examined my diet history, I realized I was the Rocky Balboa of dieters. I'd jump into the ring, boxing gloves on. "I'm ready! I can do it this time! I'm going to win this weight-loss fight no matter what. I'll set rules, strict rules. The more pressure I put on myself the better. 'No pain, no lose,' that's my dieting philosophy. No cheats, no treats, no junk. I'm going to *prove* myself. Prepare to be amazed by my discipline and willpower. I'll make it to my goal. Perfection all the way!"

Three weeks into the diet, I'm doing great, losing weight, collecting compliments, avoiding temptation. Then, a party invitation. No sweat. I can make it. I'm a fighter. Okay three cheese hors d'oeuvres and a handful of nuts—no biggie—just a sucker punch. I can handle that. A piece of garlic bread, some more cheese, a couple of glasses of wine, some more cheese, another cracker . . . "pass the chips and dip." A left hook, another punch—feeling weak. A right jab. *Come on Jen, pick yourself up*. More treats. More food. Stumble. Stagger. Sway. *I . . . can't . . . take . . . it . . .* Crash! I hit the mat. *I've blown it . . . again!*

That was my history: come out swinging, finish knocked down—defeated.

With every diet, it got harder and harder to pick myself up and get back in the ring.

Unless I figured out a new and better way to handle my weight problem or just gave up, I'd be climbing back into the ring for the rest of my life.

Dieting inflicted too many wounds: bruised confidence, battered determination, broken promises.

Jennifer, I said, *your dieting record is 0 for 25, maybe worse. Why? What are you doing wrong? You can't keep this up forever!*

I finally *had* to tell myself, *Jennifer, your boxing days are over. You have to find another way.*

Deep down, I knew what the "other way" was, I just didn't like it. I think we all know what we need to do, or we can guess. It's about changing our behaviors. It's about changing our relationship with food. It's about allowing ourselves time to make those changes. It's about allowing ourselves to make mistakes. It's about giving up perfection.

Dieting almost guarantees failure. Unless your behaviors change, it is nearly impossible to maintain diet-produced weight loss. Statistics prove it. That's because diets focus on the diet only. They encourage us to concentrate on beginning the diet and ending it. They never provide a realistic *long-term* plan to follow. They are a temporary vehicle that was never constructed to carry us through life.

Okay, let's pretend you're someone who wants to cross the ocean. You build a long, huge platform that extends out, over the water. At the top of that platform you climb onto your bicycle. Pedaling as fast as you can, you fly down that platform until you reach the end, at which point you become airborne. You're soaring! . . . Until you hit the water. Then you sink. Frantic for air, fighting the current, you struggle back to shore. "I failed again," you tell to yourself. "Why can't I reach my goal?"

The fact is, you're trying to reach your goal on a bicycle (that's the diet) while the other people who want to cross the ocean are doing it in a boat! They're using a vehicle designed for the job. Would you choose a *bicycle* to cross the ocean? Why choose a *diet* to change your life?

As a dieter, I never asked myself, "Even if I lose weight, how will I keep it off?" I never wanted to think about *permanent* life changes. We dieters spend much of the time afraid. We fear self-sabotage. We don't trust ourselves.

Remember, you haven't failed yourself. You've simply been using the wrong approach to reach your goal.

I always hated starting a diet. I hated the weighing, measuring and the food restrictions. I didn't like eating differently than everyone else. I was always afraid I wouldn't get enough to eat. I also lived with the fear that I'd fail.

Some diets were like science projects, difficult to follow and time consuming. They often required both physical and mental preparation. The diet provided a focus, but in the wrong area. I should have been focusing on *why* I was eating the way I was eating. Instead, diets provided a distraction. They encouraged me to think about controlling food, not about changing my unhealthy relationship with food.

I never thought about what I would do once I reached my ideal size. I had a more immediate focus: a project to organize. My diet survival strategy: "Just make it through today."

It was time to make a major change in the way I approached weight loss. I had to let go of "totally in control/totally out of control." If it existed, I was determined to find a realistic middle ground.

Instinct told me I had made the right decision. My new weight-loss approach *would* take time, but that was okay. *Fast* was no longer my goal. *Permanent* was my new weight-loss goal. And I was willing to accept the fact that striving for perfection doesn't result in permanent.

This time I was going to lose weight *without* a diet. I wasn't going to suffer, give up my favorite foods, or make endless lists of foods that were off limits. *I* was going to make *me* the priority, not the diet.

To a chronic dieter, this non-diet approach to weight loss sounds impossible. But I was determined to learn from my mistakes. I was determined to change my life, and at last become the person I knew I could be.

Failing with an A+

I was either an A+ diet student or a solid F. Through sessions with my clients, I've discovered most chronic dieters are this way.

When we're dieting we have to be perfect. I always followed a new diet to the letter. If I didn't, I was a failure.

No no, shouldn't have a cookie. Uh-oh, had a cookie. Bad move. Cookie bad. Cookie not on "okay-to-eat list." Shame on me. I'm bad. I've failed. Might as well eat five more.

A decision like that isn't based on logic. It's the process of jumping from the "perfect/in control" mind-set to "I've failed so I might as well give up." It's black or white thinking.

Like the old, dieting me, most of my clients (the diet perfectionists) allow no gray area. Their judgments are always black or white. Complete control of what they eat is always the major weight-loss issue.

This is why we ultimately fail. We convince ourselves again that we're ready to "do it," only to realize again that we're lacking the willpower and strength needed to be perfect all the time.

Perfection requires all our energy. That's why we wait for that ideal time to begin a diet—a time when there are no major issues going on in our lives and few distractions. But that never lasts. Something always provides a complication: a vacation, holiday parties, family problems. Then we panic. This wasn't supposed to happen. The next thing we know our ability to keep our diet-focus is gone.

Beginning a diet is like taking control of a train. The diet is the track. Every dieter is an engineer. In control, heading toward a weight goal, traveling a perfectly straight course. We want desperately to make it to our destination without hitting a single bump on the way.

Then it happens: we eat three slices of pizza, and later at the movies, a large popcorn and some candy. Uh oh! Our diet train is bumping, leaning hard to the right. This train trip is no longer perfect, no longer that absolutely straight and steady course. We feel guilty about the popcorn, pizza, and candy. *What the hell? I'm eating some cookies, and more junk.* Now our diet train is out of control. There's no hope of getting it back on course. The train flies off the tracks, flips over, and slides down the embankment. Crash. Boom. We're derailed. The diet's over.

Sound familiar?

Now, imagine a different track, a realistic track. It's built with curves and bends. True, mistakes produce bumps in the ride, but the track can still lead us to our destination. We can handle the curves and bends. The key: *we don't have to derail.*

Again we eat pizza, candy and buttered popcorn. We're upset because—let's face it—guilt comes with making bad food choices while you're *supposed* to be trying to lose weight. We all know eating a large buttery popcorn, candy, and pizza isn't a formula for successful weight loss. We've let ourselves down. Our weight loss is sabotaged. Or is it?

We've made a mistake, true, but there's no reason to give up. We haven't failed. The bad choices just represent a bump on the track—a *bump*. We don't have to *choose* to derail. Focusing on how good or bad we are is the wrong approach. Stay focused on your weight-loss *goal*, not the *ride*. Remember, it's about *reaching your destination,* not about maintaining perfection.

I stopped giving up. I stopped allowing my train to crash and burn. I was finally able to do that when I eliminated the overwhelming pressures I created by insisting that my diet journey be perfect.

I once ate four candy bars during my *successful* weight-loss train trip. Come to think of it, I once ate an entire pizza. I ate a box of chocolates. I even ate a half-gallon of ice cream in one sitting! Talk about some major bumps in the track! But I didn't allow those bumps to make me derail.

I finally accepted the truth: years of unhealthy eating behaviors were not going to be "fixed" in "diet time." I'd have to be delusional to believe I'd never again engage in out-of-control food behaviors. Hey, I enjoyed sitting in front of the TV watching my favorite shows with a container of mint chip ice cream. I cannot tell a lie.

Today, at my dream size, I still occasionally give myself a very rough train ride. But I no longer allow bad behaviors to spiral out of control. This is the hardest thing for chronic dieters to learn and accept because diets have conditioned us to operate in extremes.

People without weight problems eat ice cream. People without weight problems eat pizza. People without weight problems eat candy bars. People without weight problems don't spend their lives obsessing about food.

My final, seventy-pound, successful weight-loss train trip took about one year longer than any of my past weight-loss attempts. *But,*

by then, I had learned to accept reality; I'm human. F
cake at a birthday party (like everybody else there)
guilt trip. I've kept my weight off for over eight yea
myself to occasionally have what a strict diet-followc.
food.

Diet Cycle

I created a simple, visual tool to demonstrate why diets don't work. It
looks like this:

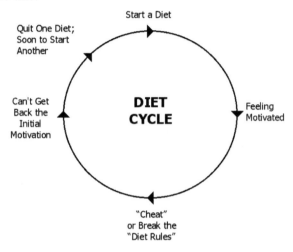

There it was in black and white: my life as a chronic dieter. I had gone
nowhere by following the same misguided cycle: losing and gaining
weight over and over again.

The diet cycle always produced the same disappointing results. It
was obvious, when I looked at the diagram, that I was on a path to
nowhere. Going in circles wasn't the answer, but how could I escape?

I had only two choices: I could continue to live a black-and-white
in-control/out-of-control life, or I could accept the truth.

- Reality #1: I had the power to change my life.
- Reality #2: I was not going to solve my food issues through
  diets. No more diets for me—ever.

Whew! What a relief!

No matter what I did, no matter how badly I messed up, no matter
what I ate, I would keep moving toward my goal. **I would not let
myself get discouraged.** Reaching my goal became the most important thing in my life.

As long as I was moving forward—not going in circles—I knew I would eventually succeed.

This was a brand-new attitude for me. For the first time, I was actually excited and confident about losing weight. Have you ever felt excited and completely stress free when you thought about weight loss?

I can tell you to give up on perfection and control, but don't expect to do it overnight. I didn't.

After successfully maintaining my weight loss for about three years I was still in the process of changing my behaviors. I was still challenging myself, because I hadn't learned to completely trust myself around food.

Dinner was one hour away. I was bored. I wanted a snack. I spotted a huge can of chocolate chips sitting on my mom's counter. They called to me. I opened the can. I started by eating just a few, but soon began to stuff huge handfuls into my mouth.

"What are you doing, Jennifer? Dinner is in an hour."

"Mom, leave me alone, I can't stop . . . I'm out of control!"

Her response confused me. *"No, you're not."*

No, you're not? Her reaction made me stop and think. I had just labeled myself "out of control." That gave me permission to head straight for the "numb zone," that place in my head where I could eat as much as I wanted without thinking about it. As long as I was *there* I could hide from guilt. Of course it would all catch up with me later. It always did. I'd look back in disgust at what I had done, beat myself up, and demand unrealistic promises from myself regarding *all* eating behaviors in the future. But while I was in that out-of-control mode, I didn't have to worry about that. Guilt was on hold.

When I was intent on overeating, I never wanted anyone to destroy my mission. This time I declared myself out of control because I *wanted* to be told to stop. This was the first time I had stopped in the middle of *choosing* to lose control.

I was flabbergasted when my mother said what she said. I had prepared myself for an attack. I was sure she would stop me, using the same language I used on myself: "What's wrong with you? You should be ashamed of yourself!" Mentally I had braced myself for the harsh judgment I was *certain* I was about to get. It was an experiment.

Overeating is usually our private little game. *How much can I get away with before anyone notices?* Deep down I knew announcing I was powerless was an excuse that supported my out-of-control behaviors.

During my heaviest days I'd sometimes engage in these behaviors with an understanding girlfriend, one who'd say something like, "I hear ya, honey. Pass those chocolate chips *my* way." We'd stuff ourselves, riding our runaway trains, intent on crashing together.

Announcing to my mom what I was preparing to do, was the first time I'd declared myself "out of control" in front of someone who *wasn't* likely to understand. *What would happen?*

*A*t the same time, I was testing myself.

The real surprise? She didn't even take my announcement seriously! Was she nuts! I had just committed a horrible food crime! I had been *bad*! Where was the guilt? Where was the criticism? She acted as though it was no big deal!

I think, at that moment, I let go of the belief that food controlled my behaviors. *I had a choice.*

I was gradually learning to accept bumps in the track, but they were still *terrifying*. Part of me didn't trust myself to get it "right." Part of me still longed for perfection. Thinking in gray felt very unnatural and uncomfortable. I was still learning that developing a middle ground does not mean surrendering to whatever happens around food. Thinking in gray simply means giving up on having to be perfect.

In the past, in my dieting days, an out-of-control "chocolate moment" would often result in destructive eating behaviors that continued through dinner, after dinner, into the following day and possibly the following week, ruining any and all weight-loss progress I had made.

During my successful weight loss, these damaging food events *still* occurred, but I was gradually learning to look at them as bumps and curves in my weight-loss train track. They were no longer the crashing, destructive, depressing *end* of my trip to my weight-loss goal. I could make bad food choices—such as pizza and buttery popcorn, and handfuls of chocolate chips—*and* engage in bad food behaviors—like eating too much at one time—and still focus on my goal. These events didn't provide an excuse to quit.

Don't let me give you the impression that destructive food behaviors no longer bother me. I still engage in them, and they still upset me. What's different? I've learned to lighten up, not be as hard on myself. I knew that stuffing chocolate morsels into my mouth wasn't healthy food behavior. Today, if someone described that behavior to me I'd say, "Don't beat yourself up. Forget about it. Keep heading toward your goal." But at the time I ate the chocolate chips, it was *still* very hard for me to stand back and look at my *own* behavior that way.

Giving Up on Perfection

Your weight-loss effort can survive a couple of handfuls of chocolate chips. But eating four handfuls becomes a deliberate act of destruction, self-punishment for choosing to eat them in the first place.

I've lost seventy pounds and kept it off, but I occasionally slip back into old behaviors. The old Jennifer (who *still* expects perfection) tries to make me feel guilty. But then, I didn't really expect her to just disappear. I will *always* have to deal with "control" issues around food. It's my nature. But I have learned to successfully negotiate with myself. I've learned to be kinder and more patient.

Food isn't "good" or "bad," it is our behaviors that undermine or support our efforts to lose weight. When we learn to control at least some of our behaviors, we lose weight and can keep it off for good.

Go, Rita, Go!

"Rita" entered my office upset and discouraged. She'd lost and regained weight throughout her life. By the time she came to me Rita was at her highest weight. "I'm out of control," she told me.

One of Rita's friends had suggested she see me. I'd lost weight and kept it off, they told her. Her friend had obviously failed to explain my weight-loss philosophy. Rita wanted a magic formula. She had no interest in taking the time to change her life.

"When can I get started?" She asked the question before she sat down.

"I need some information first," I told her. "What's your life like? Hectic? What diets have you tried in the past?"

In Rita's mind, my questions were a waste of time. After all, while we were talking she could *already* have started a diet. She could already be avoiding specific foods and planning an eating strategy.

She wanted a diet, *any* diet, immediately. Rita wanted to put a stop to her crazy eating behaviors the instant she entered my office. She wanted a solution for her food issues, and she wanted it in less than one hour. She was frantic for a program that provided strict, absolute control.

I refer to my desperate-for-control clients as "List People." They can't leave my office without a list in hand, telling them what they can and cannot eat. They want everything mapped out for them: how many calories, how many potato chips, how many slices of bread would I allow them in a day? Which foods are good, which are bad? What size apple would I allow them to eat? Does a tomato add to the calorie count? What about grapes? How do I feel about low-fat crackers? "Can I have three? How about cookies? My best friend Helen went on a 'cookie' diet and lost four pounds in a week—should I try that? How about pancakes?"

Rita and her husband go for breakfast once a week and she loves pancakes. She was sure I would tell her "no more pancakes" . . . so she had eaten seven on Sunday. "But today," she announces, "I'm ready to take strict control of my life!"

From that moment on, Rita was prepared to be perfect.

"List People" are fed-up dieters, panicked and frustrated. They have let themselves down so many times they no longer trust themselves. They are out of control and feel that they're helpless without strict guidance. They insist on having a very rigid diet plan, because that is the only way they feel *in control.*

Rita wasn't interested in examining her behaviors and changing what she was doing wrong. She wanted me to motivate her while she tried what she assumed would be another extreme approach to weight loss.

She told me she was prepared to "hit the gym" five days a week. On Saturdays she planned to go in the morning *and* evening. She had already warned her family. "Mommy will be very different for the next few weeks."

I suspect Rita thought I would be impressed. She was thoroughly dedicated; a woman prepared to learn it all, to follow all the rules.

I explained to Rita that we wouldn't be discussing food until *next* week. I told her I wanted her to keep eating what she normally ate until the next session, when we'd examine her eating patterns together. We would then focus on trying to break a lifetime of on-again/off-again dieting habits.

I'll never forget the look on Rita's face. It was a combination of panic and anger. How could I ask her to continue living the way she was living? How dare I waste her time! She could have used the thirty minutes she'd just spent with me dieting.

Rita and I arrived at the same conclusion: my weight-loss approach wasn't for her. She still had the I'm-ready-to-start-let's-get-going mind-set. She wanted the traditional diet tools: rules, lists, "good" and "bad" food categories.

The "Ritas" may go on dieting forever.

I understand. Remember me? I made countless weight-loss attempts before I got the courage to step back and take a hard and realistic look at what I was doing.

I *was* a "Rita." When I made the decision to lose weight, I wanted to take control that second. I know what it's like to need someone or something to provide that control. Without a list, without direction, I, too, felt helpless about my eating.

The irony is that I finally found genuine weight-loss success when I abandoned those old diet rules.

Success?

I recently gave a motivational lecture to a group of women at a health club. One woman in the audience raised her hand. She had something she was anxious to share. "I agree with your weight-loss philosophy," she said, "but I feel changing your life to lose weight is too long and difficult a process. The only time I've ever been successful was when I was on a diet program." She went on to say that the diet clinic was run by a famous Boston doctor. He had put her on a very strict plan. In just six months she had lost over eighty pounds.

She shared the doctor's name with the other sixty women in the room. Some carefully jotted it down.

Did anyone else notice this woman was at least 100 pounds overweight?

I asked her what her definition of "success" was. She answered, "A program that keeps me in control and takes the weight off fast!"

She had lost eighty pounds, gained it all back and more, but she still considered this famous doctor and his strict plan as a "successful" weight-loss experience.

Most of the other women in the room were very impressed as well. They wanted to know more about the doctor and his methods. After all, he promised the magic combination: *easy and fast.*

I was offering them behavioral changes designed to last a lifetime. *That* wasn't likely to be fast or easy.

I could see "promise me the quick fix" in their eyes. I felt discouraged. Didn't they get it? Then I remembered, it took *me* some time to "get it," too.

Ten years earlier I would have agreed with their definition of success. Fast and easy had also defined success countless times.

Genuine success means losing weight and keeping it off. To achieve success you must give yourself time to *change who you are*. If you don't, you'll be struggling endlessly with the same problems. If you focus only on food being either good or bad, you'll return to your old weight-gaining ways after every diet.

We desperately want to change our body overnight, but we know we can't. Time becomes our obsession. Every dieting attempt is supposed to be the "championship match," the one that ends our weight problems, fast and forever.

Say this out loud: I will work slowly to change old habits. I will develop good habits that will last a *lifetime.*

How do you feel when you say this? Write down your feelings. On a piece of paper, record what you think your most successful dieting attempt has been so far. What made it successful? If it "worked" why are you exploring new weight-loss options? Having read this chapter, do you have a new weight-loss success definition?

The Dreaded Scale

I don't have a scale in my office. My new clients usually have a frantic reaction to that piece of information. "Jennifer, what weight-loss business doesn't use a scale? How will I know if I'm losing weight? I've *always* relied on the scale! The scale shows me how much I'm losing and how fast I'm losing it!"

That's exactly the point. That's why I avoid the scale and I encourage my clients to do the same.

At the beginning of my successful weight loss, I was stepping on the scale an average of two times a day. When the number didn't change, I would ask myself, "What's the point? I should just give up." If the number was lower, I'd feel good and decide I could be less strict. I had room to "play" with my food choices.

In time I came to recognize that this heartless little measuring device had far too much power. It dictated how I felt about myself on a daily basis. "Good" or "bad" numbers in the morning determined how I could eat for the rest of the day. I'd sometimes deprive myself all week, and expect a significant loss. If the numbers were higher than I expected, the scale shattered my morale.

I began to realize that weighing myself *obsessively* wasn't going to help me. In fact, weighing myself that way became a damaging game. I was looking to a machine for endorsement and for criticism.

During one failed diet, I had avoided every temptation, making "perfect" choices, trying desperately to break 190 pounds. "This is it," I told myself one morning after a party. I had been "perfect." I had passed on every savory hors d'oeuvre that came my way. "I'm feeling thinner."

Preparing to weigh myself, I moved slowly toward the scale, holding onto the sink. (I always thought this helped.) Then, I carefully lowered my full weight onto the scale. "Up two pounds? How can this be? I was 'perfect' last night. I should have *lost* weight! This is ridiculous! This stinks!"

I was angry, but that quickly changed to a feeling of utter defeat, which provided a great excuse to give up. When the scale disappointed me, I almost always used that disappointment to justify spending the rest of the day eating what I wanted, whenever I wanted it.

But, even "good" numbers can produce "bad" behaviors.

When I ate poorly and treated myself to things I knew I shouldn't have, and then the numbers indicated that I hadn't gained, I developed a hey-I-can-get-away-with-more-than-I-thought! attitude.

The scale always creates a no-win situation. As a result, I had a love/hate relationship with it. Mostly *hate*. It surprised me to learn that I was not the only one who hated the scale.

After I reached my final weight-loss goal, I wanted to help other people achieve their weight-loss goals as well. I took a part-time job as a motivational lecturer at a weight-loss center. My job included weighing people before they heard the weight-loss "topic of the week."

Recording other people's weight was a horrible job! You would think I was leading them to their doom. Before getting on the scale, dieters, in a state of panic, offered nervous excuses for weight gain.

"I'm feeling bloated. I know I'm retaining water!"

"I had some cake last night. I'm sure I gained!"

Or, "I was perfect all week! I better have lost weight!"

The center even made a box available for people to put their belongings in. I waited while they removed earrings, rings, scarves, hair clips, pins—anything to lower their numbers. They were all frantic.

It was too much for me. I had succeeded by letting go of the perfect-or-failed approach to weight loss. These weigh-ins went against everything I had learned.

The scale can become a distraction, focusing your energy and attention in the wrong place.

One client who was a scale "shopper" confided, "The scale at the doctor's office reads four pounds heavier than the one at my house, but the scale at my health club," she added excitedly, "reads six pounds lighter! That's my favorite!"

Other clients make themselves slaves to the scale.

"Jennifer, I'm so bummed! Yesterday afternoon I was 156, this morning I'm at 158! How could that happen?"

Scale addicts don't trust themselves. Giving up the scale is traumatic because they believe they need the scale to maintain control.

The scale has a negative effect on almost every dieter. If you can *honestly* say it doesn't get to you, then go ahead, weigh yourself. But I've never met *anyone*, including me, who is unaffected by those numbers, good or bad. If weighing yourself produces bad behaviors, do yourself a favor: eliminate the scale altogether.

My clients usually resist giving up the scale at first. They don't think of it in terms of removing pressure. They see taking the scale away as a frightening change. For most of them, the scale is their *only* method of measuring success or failure. And, the more scale obsessed a client is, the less likely they are to succeed and the harder it is for me to convince them to toss the scale.

We dieters like to be held accountable in some way.

We want to see—at any given moment—that what we're doing is working. But ironically, we also go to the scale when we know we've done the *wrong* thing because it's also a source of punishment.

If you change the way you define success—losing weight and keeping it off—a short-term win is really not winning at all.

Use something other than the scale to evaluate your progress. I record my clients' progress by using a measuring tape, a "before" photo, and a body-fat test.

A body-fat test can be done at most health clubs where there's a certified fitness trainer. That person can tell you what your ideal body fat percentage should be.

If you don't feel comfortable going to a health club for this test, the "before" photo and body measurements are enough. It was some time before I mustered the courage to get a body-fat test. I was terrified of exposing myself to my polar opposite. What would they think?

It wasn't until I had dropped three sizes that I let some hard-bodied fitness-nut pinch my rolls. Even then, it was difficult to put my less-than-ideal body in a vulnerable situation. But I focused on my goal. What was more important, what some stranger thought of my body or my weight-loss success?

As a rule, I record my clients' weight-loss progress monthly. I use a cloth measuring tape to measure the top of the biceps (upper arm), waist (where the pants waistline rests), hips (at the widest point), and the upper thigh. I use calipers to measure body fat percentages. I "pinch" the front and back of the upper arm, the upper back, and the stomach. For the perfectionist eager to see progress, evaluating changes by measuring on a monthly basis is a lesson in patience.

When clients agree to accept my once-a-month time frame, they discover that this approach removes a lot of pressure. For us perfectionists, less pressure results in less panic. Less panic gives us the freedom to examine our eating behaviors and change them.

Unfortunately, the scale anchors us in a zone where only "perfect" or "horrible" is measured. Stepping away from the scale moves us closer to that balanced, gray area from which we need to learn to operate.

In the process of weight loss, a mistake does not have to result in failure and attempting perfection will *not* produce success.

Often, having more time between evaluations of their progress is a luxury for my clients. "Jennifer, the measuring tape isn't as gratifying as the scale. I used to like seeing those numbers go down," one client put it. "But I enjoy focusing on the changes in my body. I can see I'm losing weight, and I feel terrific."

One of my favorite ways of measuring my weight-loss progress was with my clothes. Feeling my clothes getting baggy was more exciting than stepping on the scale! As my favorite pair of pants got looser and looser, I became increasingly more confident.

How you *look and feel* is what matters most.

Pick your dream size. Take your measurements. Work towards a "size goal." That works for my clients. It worked for me. And it can work for you, too.

One Small Step—One Big Change

When I made the commitment to lose weight the right way, I decided that no one food would be off limits. I could have foods I loved, but I would have to learn how to eat them in a healthy way. I wanted to lose weight, but like other people, I wanted my favorite foods, too.

I wasn't prepared to give up anything for a lifetime. Every time I tried the no-more-of-that approach, it backfired. "No more sugar, Jennifer! It's the root of all your weight problems. If you don't eat sugar, you will be thin."

My no-sugar promise lasted only until finally I broke down and had some of the forbidden treat. Then, all hell broke loose. I even put sugar on french fries! For me, putting anything off limits was asking for trouble.

Telling myself I couldn't have something I loved made that food even more appealing and desirable. It was just a matter of time before I went back to my off-limits food and made up for the time we'd been apart. It was a sick and destructive love affair.

I needed a new, healthier and realistic strategy.

At the time I was preparing to begin my final, permanent weight loss, my every weekend treat was a large box of incredibly delicious fried clams. I'd eat them until I was stuffed, feeling sick.

I'd made a commitment to lose weight in a new way, but I couldn't bear the thought of giving up my fried clams.

What could I do?

"What's your smallest portion?" I asked the woman at the clam stand. She pulled an itty-bitty white box up from under the counter. I cringed. I hadn't known a box that small existed. Who in their right mind would choose that size? I was on the verge of panic, but I stopped myself. Which was more important: the clams or my weight-loss goal?

I'd made a commitment to me, and a new life. This was my chance, an opportunity to take my very first, small, positive behavioral step. I'd already accepted that I'd have food issues for life; there was no cure. I'd given up on diets and setting time limits. Now it was time to prove to myself that I could eat what I had always labeled "non-diet" food in a way that would still allow me to lose weight.

I ordered what they called the appetizer size. Usually I like to see a lot of food on my plate. So, to keep myself from feeling deprived, I took the clams home. I made a big salad and ate it with the clams. The salad helped me adjust to the small clam serving. I savored every last bite.

I'm not going to tell you I was thrilled about the tiny clam portion, but at least the clams were there. I got to taste them, to enjoy them, and I didn't spend time obsessing about the fact that they were off limits, which is what the old "dieting me" had always done.

When I finished the clam meal, I felt proud of my accomplishment. I had a right to feel proud. I had taken my first food step toward success.

You might think ordering *anything* fried while trying to lose weight was a bad idea. But that's the familiar and flawed all-or-nothing way of looking at weight loss. I would never have believed it, but my infant-size portion (combined with the huge salad piled on my plate) satisfied me!

Making the food you love best the smallest portion on your plate and bulking it up with non-trigger foods (usually fruits or vegetables) will help you adjust to a new way of eating. The main issue for me was volume. As long as I could look at my plate and see a lot of food, I didn't panic.

I'd learned my most important weight-loss lesson: I could eat the things I loved if I ate them in a different way. My feeling of accomplishment made it much easier to order the appetizer-size next time.

Okay, I know what you're thinking. You're thinking the same thing many of my clients tell me: "Jen, I can't eat just one small portion of my favorite food! Impossible!"

Don't assume you *have* to lead yourself into frantic eating behaviors.

Thoughtfully, calmly, consider the alternative.

In my experience, almost everyone with food issues engages in the same behaviors. When the former dieting-Jennifer visited the clam bar, she panicked. *I'm not supposed to be here! This is a mistake, but I have to have the taste of fried clams. I'll get the super size and get this over with.*

I'd order the largest size and eat until I felt ill, having to undo the top button of my pants. *That's the last time I'll be eating those for awhile!* I'd convince myself that I'd gotten the taste of fried clams out of my system. *Now*, I told myself, *I'm prepared to stay in control. From now on I'll be perfect.*

Try to imagine yourself buying the smallest serving size. You may be thinking, *I can't do that!* You're thinking about experiencing a level of satisfaction, not about hunger. We know that a small box of clams, a huge salad, and a piece of fruit will fill us up, but this isn't about getting enough to eat, it's about getting enough of a specific taste.

I've noticed that when I eat something I feel guilty about, I don't really taste anything beyond the first bite. I may inhale two pounds of it, but I don't savor it, or enjoy it. I taste the first cookie. I don't taste the next six.

Consider how you eat the foods that make you feel guilty.

Commonly, when we make a decision to be "bad" we go all the way. But when I chose to order my first small serving of clams I was determined not to feel guilty about eating something I loved. I had made a *choice* to eat a small amount of something that, in my dieting past would have been labeled "forbidden." This time I didn't just give up control and surrender to a temptation—I made a conscious decision. For the very first time I was telling myself that eating a *reasonable* serving of clams was okay. That decision—choosing to eat my favorite foods in a moderate way—was one of the hardest things I ever did.

For us, it's "*all* or nothing," never "*small* or none."

Ten years ago, my food choices and habits were driven by fear, not reality. I was afraid I wouldn't get enough if I ate less. I was afraid I wouldn't be satisfied after eating a small serving. I was afraid of a "life" change. I was afraid that anything other than dieting the old way wouldn't work. But I eventually proved that *moderation* is the only thing that does work.

Those of us who diet chronically are not willing to live in a state of misery and deprivation indefinitely. Why should we? But we are not happy living in bodies we hate. Why should we be? Unfortunately, we assume it has to be one choice or the other. It doesn't.

That first step toward changing your behaviors requires courage.

Name your most forbidden food, the one that's most likely to produce out-of-control behavior. Name it out loud.

Purchase that food and have a small portion of it. If it's pizza, for example, buy an individual slice. Is it candy? Buy a small amount, eat half. French fries? Order a small serving, eat all but the last few. It will become easier each time you successfully do it. Discovering you don't have to surrender your power to food is exciting. It's an empowering experience.

3

New Habits, New Body

Who, Me?

For much of my young adult life, I weighed over two hundred pounds. I could claim a rare, metabolic disorder (acquired from a bacteria-contaminated sticky bun) caused my obesity. I could tell you I spent my overweight life eating small portions of healthy food, but—to the shock of the medical world—my fat cells continued to expand. "How can this be?" medical specialists asked. Scientists from all over the world begged to study me.

I wish I *could* tell you this story. I wish it were true, then I wouldn't have to take responsibility for my body. The painful truth? I ate too much and moved too little.

Because we feel frustrated and desperate some of us find just about any explanation for weight gain—even a health related one—less embarrassing than confronting our dysfunctional relationship with food.

Not every dieter looks at his or her weight problem this way, but I did.

As a child, I had been very sick and lost a lot of weight. I became very frail. When I finally began to recover from my illness, I ate non-stop. After overhearing my mother explain my childhood illness to a friend, I used that story to provide a reason for my overeating and weight gain.

47

At six years old, my illness excuse made some sense. Fifteen years later, it started sounding a little old: "And my mommy said that I got soooo sick, I wanted lots and lots of food. . . ."

My childhood illness may have been a legitimate reason for weight gain for a short time after I recovered. But fifteen years later, *even I* didn't believe that excuse any more. Still, it gave me an explanation for my out-of-control food behaviors and my failed dieting attempts.

I'd start diet after diet full of hope and always end up disappointed and defeated. My failures *had* to be my fault. The diets *promised* effortless success. It wasn't the diet I blamed for my weight-loss failure: I blamed myself for not being able to stick to the diet. After failing on the diet, I'd fall back on my old illness story. Maybe *that* diet worked for *other* people, but since it didn't work for *me*, my condition must be unique. Wasn't it possible that as a result of my childhood illness I had a malfunctioning metabolism?

The truth? Diets, particularly fad diets, don't work long-term for *anybody*. Take my word for it. As a weight-loss coach, I hear the *real* stories, the feelings of frustration and disappointment, the sense of failure these diets produce. The only weight-loss approach that *will* change your life is *you* taking responsibility for, and changing, your eating behaviors.

Don't confuse taking responsibility with assuming blame. We *blame* food allergies for our weight gain. We *blame* our bodies, believing they fail us by processing food in a faulty way. We *blame* our choice of diets. "If only I'd found the *right* diet, I'd have been able to stick with it!" We blame those food allergies, our genes, our diet choices, because we think that if we don't blame other things, our only choice is to blame ourselves. Blame, of *any* kind, is destructive, painful, and pretty much guarantees our repeated weight-loss failures.

Blame is negative; it's about guilt. It drives us into frantic behaviors and unrealistic solutions for our weight problem. Blame is frightening, but accepting responsibility, without guilt, isn't.

When I suggest to you that *you have* to take responsibility for your eating behaviors, I'm not suggesting that your behaviors are "bad." Blame is about bad. Blame is about judgments. Blame is about being ashamed. Blame won't get you where you want to go: taking responsibility will.

There is *nothing* wrong with you, you just have a problem you want to solve, and you're ready to do that, *right*?

It's that simple. If you were wearing a coat that was too warm, you wouldn't continue to wear it, sweating, while you walked around, day after day, telling yourself, "It's the manufacturer's fault. They should never have made a coat *this* heavy! It's the store's fault. They should never have sold me a coat *this* warm!" You would simply say, "Gosh, I'm too warm in this coat. I think I'll take it off."

For those of us who are angry or disappointed with ourselves, taking responsibility can feel like making ourselves the target for our own anger. It feels less painful to make other things the target.

Instead of spending valuable time looking for reasons or excuses for weight gain, spend your time productively, making positive and healthy changes in your life. You deserve much more than just finding excuses for being overweight.

"I'm following your advice but I'm not losing weight. You don't understand, ever since I was abducted by aliens. . . ."

Okay, maybe I haven't heard *this* excuse, but I've heard plenty of them that are equally unrealistic. My point is that when the excuse for being overweight becomes more important than weight loss, I know that client isn't ready.

My weight-loss business is 95 percent motivational. I motivate people to do the things they *can* do in order to be healthy, things they're already aware of, but don't have enough faith in themselves to do.

If you can distinguish the difference between *blame* and *responsibility*, you're already on your way to success!

Please, Please Don't Make Me Count Calories!

This section of the book was difficult to write. I don't want to encourage you to become obsessive about fat grams, food labels, or portions. Since you're reading this book, I guarantee that you've already obsessed about at least one of these food-related issues. I don't want you to ever do that again. But, I couldn't leave the topic of food out of this book all together.

You're entitled to expect some basic, food-related information. Much of that information is available to you through books that have a healthy eating and nutrition focus. You can find most of those books at the library. I've read many of them and, in addition, have taken several nutrition and weight-management courses. I acquired much practical information through personal experiences, as well as those shared by my clients. You may already know some of this information. Some of it you may never have thought about. I *can* promise that if you take the information in this section—new and old—and apply it to your life, it will help you reach your goal.

If you want to broaden your knowledge of nutrition (which I recommend you do), read books focused on healthy food choices, *not* books with a diet focus.

Generally, we know what we *should* and *should not* be eating. We might not know the chemical breakdown of a cupcake, but we know that if given the choice between an apple and a cupcake, we *should* choose the apple. If you're trying to lose weight, eating two slices of pizza makes more sense than eating four. A huge cheeseburger or a salad with grilled chicken? Let's see . . . which one would be the better choice? Bing, bing, bing . . . you win! (You *did* choose the salad with chicken, right?)

We chronic dieters (current and former) are far from clueless, but unfortunately, there are plenty of bogus diet salespeople who treat us as if we were. If we're guilty of anything, it may be that we're too trusting! Diet book authors continue to give us the same old repackaged information, with the promise that it's *new,* and we continue to *believe* them!

Weight loss is *always* connected to calorie reduction. Fad diet books disguise this basic fact by wrapping it in pseudo-scientific jargon and filler. Often, in the time it takes us to finish one of these books, we could have taken a nutrition course at a hospital, a course that would teach us gimmick-free, sensible skills that we could use for life.

This section of the book won't tell you exactly what to eat. Instead, it will help you *develop systems* that provide a healthy lifestyle, no matter what eating challenges life brings.

I will show you what I focused on while I was losing weight and outline the changes I made in my life. I will demonstrate how those changes became successful, healthy habits.

When I first developed my business, I couldn't wait to share the nutrition information I'd learned. Some of that information covered high-calorie foods, high-fat foods, the evils of fried foods, and what a realistic portion size looked like. I learned about suggested intake of vitamins and minerals and the variety of foods we should eat to maintain good health.

I was prepared to teach the world how to eat for good health and weight loss. Weren't people clueless? Didn't they *need* someone who could tell them how much fat there is in a fast-food burger? I'd enlighten them! They needed to be told how to identify a realistic portion size! Well, I would show them—I had the charts. "They'll sure be shocked when I tell them what they need to do is eat more fruits and vegetables!"

Right?

Wrong!

"Jennifer, I know this stuff. I know what I *should* be eating! I'm frustrated because I can never last on a diet program for long. Please skip the lecture and tell me how you learned to stop eating. How do you stop before you eat too much?"

Boy, was I surprised! My clients already knew much of the information I was prepared to give them!

The frustrated dieters who came to me knew *what* they should be doing. What they wanted me to share with them was *how: How* had I lost weight? *How* had I kept the weight off for so many years? *How* did I find the motivation to make it last, the willpower to stay slim? What are the *other* factors—the nonfood factors—that influenced weight-loss success?

Yikes, the pressure!

Those questions required that I reexamine the focus of my business. After being overweight for so long, why had I suddenly found the will to lose weight and keep it off? I realized that healthy weight loss wasn't *just* about learning and practicing good nutrition. It was also about changing my priorities, *me* convincing *me* that my health was the most important thing in my life.

Quality of life issues can make or break you when you're trying to lose weight. I regularly see the following factors affecting the success of my clients:

- How do they feel about their lives?
- What creates stress in their lives and how do they deal with it?

At the time I made the decision to lose weight, *I generally liked my life,* and most importantly, in spite of the fact that I was very over-weight, *I liked myself.* True, I wasn't happy with my body, but basically, I liked who I was inside.

Self-esteem issues often dictate *how* and when we lose weight. I often started the most rigid, most unrealistic diets, when I felt worst about myself, when I felt as though I'd hit rock bottom. Once, when I was in one of my heaviest phases and felt miserable I told myself, *Jennifer, you're going on an all-lettuce diet. Nothing but lettuce for one week!* The more punishing the diet, the more determined I felt when I started it. I *blamed* myself for eating bad food, and not being able to stop. I have to admit it, when I was disgusted with myself I enjoyed being mean to myself.

The *blaming* part of me liked the I'll-show-the-out-of-control-me-who's-in-charge approach to weight loss. Putting rigid food boundaries in place felt like establishing control. In reality, it just set me up for failure, but in the meantime, I was prepared to suffer.

No one should suffer while losing weight. When you *like yourself*, suffering isn't an option. Think of weight loss as a personal challenge. As a human being, you are not designed to suffer; you are designed to grow emotionally, and expand personally in self-awareness. **Weight loss is not punishment; it's a wonderful and exciting experience that will lead you to a new life**.

At the time I started my successful and final weight loss, my stress level was manageable. There was no problem in my life that created overwhelming stress.

Ironically, I've observed that clients who already have high levels of stress in their life often approach their weight loss demanding perfection of themselves, which just adds additional stress.

Nobody's life is perfect. We all have stress. At the time I began my weight loss, there were things I would have changed, but I did not have any deep-rooted stress issues that I expected weight loss to solve. If you feel you have damaging circumstances affecting your quality of life, I suggest you address them with a therapist *before* attempting weight loss.

Are you a fundamentally happy person? If you are, it's likely that food presents a small obstacle in your weight-loss process. Determination and will—driven by self-esteem—dictate who will succeed at weight loss.

Okay, we've avoided them long enough. It's time to talk about those dreaded calories.

Every teacher in every nutrition class I ever took agreed, "There is no magic formula for losing weight." They told me things I expected to hear: healthy weight loss and its maintenance is about calorie reduction, balanced eating, and exercise.

Magic formulas repeatedly get us chronic dieters into trouble! Remember that weight loss is about overall calorie reduction. Yet, some of those tricky, fad diet books would have you believe that calories have little to do with weight loss.

Would *you* stand in line to buy a diet book called *Count Calories for Life*? Probably not. Why? Boring! Besides you already know that reducing the number of calories you consume will result in weight loss.

The fad, formula diet book authors are very careful not to focus on boring, old calories. Instead they give you new, detailed instructions to follow: three ounces of *this*, mix *this* with a certain number of *that*. Shhhhh, the formula is the secret—the magic answer we've all been searching for!

The writers of these diet books tiptoe around the subject of those pesky old calories because it's stuff we already know. They keep their approach to weight loss exciting. "Not nearly enough protein in your diet," or "Naughty, naughty, you're combining foods that should never be eaten together." "You can eat from 'this' list but avoid 'that' list" and on and on. I call it busy work. It provides a distraction, so you don't notice that what they've actually done is reduced your total caloric intake.

Accept the fact that somehow, in some way, weight-loss formula diets will *always* be about calorie reduction.

Hey, I've been there! I loved busy work. I was thrilled to focus on the formula approach. "Is that red pepper I see in your sauce? Sorry Aunt Jane, I'm not allowed red pepper! Too much sugar in a *red* pepper!" "Oh, sorry Aunt Bettie, I can't eat a tomato with a starch. I'll have to pass on your pasta dish. I've recently read that tomato acid combined with wheat causes a fat cell explosion."

Having a focus makes dieting more tolerable. It feels more scientific—more structured—which makes us feel more in control.

Before my weight loss, I loved to spout diet book jargon. "I mustn't eat those crackers; white flour makes me swell." The *real* story? Three servings of *anything*, in addition to too many calories in your day, will make you swell. Being able to put the blame on food combinations made me feel different, as if what happened to *me* was unique.

I knew I was eating twice, sometimes three times what I needed, but who wants to confront that? It's a harsh and painful reality, especially when it feels like blame and you see no way to change it. But I was so miserable, I knew I had to start somewhere.

Common sense told me I should start paying attention to *exactly* what I was eating, at *all* times. I bought a book that listed the calories and fat grams of all foods and in a notebook began to record what I ate. (Sometimes a guess, considering that not all food is labeled.)

At that point, I promised myself not to change *how* I ate. I simply wanted to see what a "calorie day in the life of Jennifer" added up to. I promised myself that I would record the good, the bad, and the ugly. If I ate a bag of chips, if I ate seven of my favorite cookies, if I ate a pint of ice cream, I would record how many calories these foods provided. I would no longer live in denial. I *knew* I ate too much, but *how much* did I *really* eat?

Counting calories and recording what I ate was an eye-opening experience. While I did have "light" eating days—days where I didn't overeat or ate mostly healthy foods—I soon discovered that more "bad" days canceled out the all-too-rare "good" eating days. For every healthy day, there were countless unhealthy eating days. I wanted to tear the record of them out of the notebook and burn and destroy the evidence. It took a lot of guts to confront my eating patterns, but I knew I had to take responsibility for *everything* I ate. Was I eating 2,500 calories a day, 3,500 calories a day? Truthfully recording my eating habits and being honest with myself was the first very important step in bringing my eating under control.

I had spent a lot of time trying to figure out *why* I was overweight. When I had a healthy eating day I remembered *those* days. I'd say, "Jennifer, you've been eating so well! I can't believe you haven't been losing weight!" But when I had an eat-whatever-whenever-day, it just seemed to get erased from my memory. Conveniently forgetting the binge days, I developed a poor-me attitude.

It's easy to do, because often when we're on an eating mission, we're not thinking about what were doing.

By recording my food intake, I discovered I ate in a healthy way about twenty percent of the time.

When I recorded my calorie intake for a typical day, I discovered I was consuming around 2,500+ calories. I knew it wouldn't be realistic for me to reduce too much, too soon. Based on past experience I knew if I tried that, I'd eventually go into deprivation mode, and (when I couldn't take it anymore) I'd end up eating twice as much as *before* I'd made the weight-loss attempt.

By trial and error I gradually determined how many calories I needed per day to avoid deprivation mode. I observed a pattern. On 1,500 or less calories, I'd go to bed thinking about my next meal, unable to sleep because I felt so deprived. For me, consumption of less than 1,500 calories per day was impossible to live with. I could manage for a few weeks then I'd break down and rebelliously eat all the calories I'd "saved," cancelling out all of my hard work.

At 1,600–1,800 calories per day, I was a satisfied, happy camper. I wasn't suffering at all. Aiming for 1,600, but allowing myself up to 1,800 calories gave me a few "extra calorie" days—those days when I craved a candy bar, or a cookie, or a few pieces of cheese, like any "normal" person.

Because I allowed myself up to 1,800 calories a day, there was little reason for failure due to deprivation. My attitude was positive. *I can manage this!* I told myself. I had begun to replace my extreme approach to weight loss with a balanced approach. By providing myself with a realistic calorie allowance, I could keep my hunger meter out of the extreme range. This approach didn't involve suffering. No more counting blocks of cheese in order to fall asleep! I felt comfortable. For the first time in my life, I wasn't obsessing about food.

I'll bet I can guess what you're thinking. *Sixteen hundred calories a day? I'd never lose weight on 1,600 calories!* I'm not suggesting you use *my* numbers. I'm recommending that you arrive at your own realistic calorie range—a range that reduces your current caloric intake, but won't set you up for failure.

Experiment. Record what you've been eating and determine your *honest*, current daily calorie intake. Like me, you may be eating more than you realized, so, *any* calorie reduction—especially one you can live with—is going to have a positive effect and result in weight loss.

My client "Jake" asked me how many calories I would "allow" him in a day. I told him that because he was an avid exerciser, I felt 2,200 calories would keep him satisfied. "Wow! That's generous, Jennifer! I was sure I'd have to eat under 1,300 to lose weight."

Jake, a man standing six feet two, believed he had to eat like a small child! *Would* he lose weight on 1,300 calories? Yes. Could he keep it off? No. "Lose fast/regain fast" had been Jake's weight-loss history. He operated in extremes. He would put himself on starvation-level calories and lose weight fast. Then—because he was miserable—he'd begin his new, "thin" life by eating three times the calories per day than he'd eaten before the diet!

Healthy, fit people do not starve themselves to stay that way.

For chronic dieters, weight loss equals punishment. This should be our bumper sticker. Unless we dieters are suffering, we don't feel we're dealing with our weight problem. Jake was uncomfortable when I suggested he could lose weight on 2,200 calories per day. "Too many," was his initial reaction. Amazingly, Jake *never* felt uncomfortable about eating a whopping 3,800 calories when he went off a diet! Jake, like most dieters, was most comfortable operating in the extreme.

While examining her food diary my client "Debbie" and I discovered a pattern that was interesting. On Monday, she had eaten a piece of cake. Next to the word cake, to explain the reason she ate it (my clients often feel obliged to do this, although I don't expect them to), it said "son's birthday." On Tuesday, she ate two pieces of leftover cake. On Wednesday, she ate more cake, including the two "slivers" that "finished it off."

Debbie's behavior is a classic example of why we ultimately fail at weight loss. *One* slice of cake *would not* keep Debbie from losing weight. If Debbie continued to watch her total calorie intake for that day, she would still make weight-loss progress. *One* slice of cake was not going to slow her down. But, because Debbie focused *only* on the cake, labeling it "bad" food, she had convinced herself she had already failed.

I suggested she look at the cake incident differently. One regular-size slice of birthday cake averages about 250 calories. Not a problem. But two to three slices? Now we're getting into trouble. By getting frustrated with herself—*before* she actually had a problem—Debbie ended up eating 500 to 750 additional I-give-up-I've-failed cake calories.

I identified with my client Debbie's behavior. In the past, I had many I-blew-it days. This is how I used to eat. (Brace yourself, it's a bit scary!)

My typical day started with a poor breakfast, never balanced. It was high-fat, "on the run," or none at all. Lunch was often a large sub or a high-fat cold cut sandwich, with a big bag of chips. Dinner was often pizza. At the end of one of those "bad" food days, I'd typically develop a what-the-hell attitude. "After all," I'd say to myself, "this day is already a total food disaster. I've *already* let myself down. I'm feeling miserable after eating all that junk. I might as well go all the way and finish the day with a huge bowl of ice cream."

Recognize the all-or-nothing syndrome at work?

Maybe this eating style doesn't sound like yours. Maybe you're one of those people who doesn't eat large meals, but picks throughout the day. Maybe you don't eat junk but just too many so-called "healthy," low-fat things. Personally, I was more of a garbage-eater but for some of my clients, that's never been part of their problem. They just eat too much—even if their choices are low fat—and they move too little. Too many calories, regardless of what *kind* of calories, and little or no exercise, *will* result in weight gain.

To lose weight safely, my nutrition teachers suggested that the typical healthy woman should eat approximately 25–35 grams of fat a day (20 percent to 30 percent of total daily calories) and 1,500–1,800 calories (depending on amount of exercise). A man should eat, on average, 40–50 grams of fat a day and 1,700–2,500 calories to achieve healthy weight loss. *His or her size and activity level are factors that have to be taken into consideration. (See a nutritionist or dietitian to determine the level that is safe and realistic for you.)*

I'm a cracker lover. Often, I would open a box of my favorite crackers (intending to eat one or two) and end up polishing off the entire box. My nutrition teachers stressed that no favorite foods should be off limits. Instead, they encouraged us to determine the number of total calories we consume when we stuff ourselves with a favorite snack food, such as crackers. I learned to check labels before I started snacking to see how many calories and fat grams the typical box of crackers contained. Eventually, I learned by label reading where *all* foods fit into my life. I could eat *everything* I loved as long as I took the number of total calories and grams of fat into consideration.

Yeah, yeah, I know, you *already* read labels. That's what my clients always tell me. "I know what I should be looking for, Jennifer."

The question is how do you make the label information work for you?

When I'm teaching my clients the basics of label reading, I use product packages. One is an empty (elves ate them) cookie box. When I hold up the cookie box to show them the label, they *always* cringe. "Oh, Jennifer, I *know* how terrible those are!" They're prepared to be told, "No more of these. These cookies are very *bad*, high in fat and calories!"

But, to their surprise that's not what I say. Instead, I ask them how many cookies they would typically eat at a time. Their answer is usually four or more.

Two cookies have, on average, 160 calories and 7 grams of fat. Nutritious? Not really. Destructive? Not at that point. Two cookies won't make or break your weight-loss attempt. That's the key. I know, I know. You're out of control when you eat things you feel are bad. You wish you could have the discipline to eat only two cookies. If you stopped at eating only two, you wouldn't have a weight problem. But let's examine your choices: eat all or none, or *change your behaviors around food.* Consider a middle ground choice. With both the all-or-none choices you ultimately suffer. Choose not to suffer. Choose moderation.

Last night after dinner, I had two chocolate-drenched cookies. They were big, they were rich, and they were delicious. When I shared with a client the fact that I had indulged in the cookies, she was frustrated by my story. "How did you stop at two, Jennifer?"

I wasn't particularly proud of the fact that I'd had two! I was mad at myself for not stopping at one! (That wanting to be perfect will *always* be a part of me!) But my client's question put things into perspective. In the past, before I changed my behaviors, I would have eaten six cookies. Eating only two demonstrated that, over time, I've learned to control my behavior. *Any* reduction in what I ate would still support my effort to maintain my lost weight. My client, like me, was still hung up on that *all-or-nothing* mind-set. We need to learn, and keep reminding ourselves, that normal eating isn't about being perfect, it's about allowing ourselves to make the balanced choice.

Back to Basics

I learned to pay attention to four things.

1. **Servings per container.** Yeah, right. Maybe if I was five years old I could make a small box of crackers provide ten servings. Who are they kidding?
2. **Serving size.** Ha! A serving size from a box of my favorite crackers is four crackers? Who decides these things, a munchkin from the *Wizard of Oz*?
3. **Calories per serving.** Wow! Four crackers, 130 calories. Gee, I wonder why I had a weight problem: a typical snack was half of the box!
4. **Total fat.** Four crackers (one serving) equals 5 grams of fat. I'd have four servings (4 x 5 = 20 grams of fat). A typical snack nearly wiped out my total fat allowance for the entire day!

If you want to take this to a higher level, make an appointment with a nutritionist or dietitian to see what other things you should focus on for good health. To keep this simple, I'm just focusing on basic label information.

I knew I would have to adjust to eating a lower-calorie, lower-fat, healthier diet. This was my first goal. At the deli, I compared my favorite brand of bologna with other types on the market. While I was at it, I checked all the sandwich trimmings as well. Here is what I learned about my sandwich:

Three pieces of regular bologna:

> **270** calories
>
> **24** grams of fat

Two slices of regular cheese:

> **140** calories
>
> **10** grams of fat

One tablespoon of regular mayonnaise:
> **110** calories
> **12** grams of fat

One small bag of chips:
> **240** calories
> **14** grams of fat

Two slices of bread:
> **160** calories
> **1.5** grams of fat

My favorite sandwich and chips? A grand total of . . . **920** calories and **61.5** grams of fat!

Remember that the nutrition courses I took recommended, on average, a woman should consume approximately 35 grams of fat, a man no more than 50 per day.

I wasn't prepared to give up my favorite sandwich, but I had to explore my alternatives. Never did I consider the amount of calories and fat I was getting from one sandwich and a bag of chips.

So, I compared the low-fat numbers.

Three slices of fat-free bologna:
> **60** calories
> **0** grams of fat

One slice of fat-free cheese and one slice of regular (for flavor):
> **105** calories
> **6** grams of fat

One tablespoon of low-fat mayonnaise:
> **50** calories
> **3.5** grams of fat

One serving of *baked* potato chips:
> **110** calories
> **1.5** grams of fat

Two slices of bread:
> **160** calories
> **1.5** grams of fat.

A grand total of . . . **485** calories and **12.5** grams of fat! I saved **435** calories and **49** grams of fat!

Okay, I'll admit that I didn't jump up and down when I first tried a fat-free bologna, low-fat cheese sandwich. Neither did I do a little dance when I bit into a baked potato chip. But, I was determined to make these foods work for me. They weren't *terrible*, and I had come to realize that high fat and big portions had kept me overweight. My priority was to lose weight and I was ready. I was prepared to put *me* before food.

This could be fun. I started experimenting. I played the calorie-savings game!

Two-egg omelet:
> **160** calories
>
> **12** grams of fat

Cheddar cheese, 2 oz.:
> **200** calories
>
> **16** grams of fat

Two pork sausage patties:
> **150** calories
>
> **12** grams of fat

A grand total of . . . **510** calories and **40** grams of fat. Yikes! I'd had my entire daily fat allowance by the end of breakfast!

Now, I compared the low-fat numbers:

Egg whites (sold by the carton): 1/2 carton is the equivalent of two eggs:
> **60** calories
>
> **0** grams of fat

2 oz. reduced-fat cheddar cheese:
> **110** calories
>
> **6** grams of fat

Two lean turkey sausages or veggie sausages:
> **50** calories
>
> **1.5** grams of fat

A grand total of . . . **220** calories and **7.5** grams of fat! This translates into a savings of . . . **290** calories and **32.5** grams of fat!

Remarkable! I could still have a version of my most favorite foods, and save *hundreds of calories* and *many* grams of fat.

One boxed, frozen beef patty with cheese:

(meat and cheese only)

> **400** calories
>
> **32** grams of fat

Hamburger roll:

> **230** calories
>
> **1.5** grams of fat

A grand total of . . . **630** calories and **33.5** grams of fat.

I compared the low-fat numbers:

Veggie burger (average):

> **110** calories
>
> **1.5** grams of fat

One slice of reduced-fat cheese:

> **70** calories
>
> **5** grams of fat

Hamburger roll:

> **230** calories
>
> **1.5** grams of fat

A grand total of . . . **410** calories and **8** grams of fat. A savings of . . . **220** calories and **25.5** grams of fat!

When I was invited to a cookout, I took the initiative to compare the labels of veggie hot dogs with the regular hot dogs I used to buy. By bringing my own hot dogs, I was ensuring that I would have something low-fat to eat.

Two regular hot dogs:

> **380** calories
>
> **34** grams of fat

Two hot dog rolls:

> **220** calories
>
> **3** grams of fat

A total of . . . **600** calories and **37** grams of fat.

I compared the low-fat numbers:

Two low-fat hot dogs or veggie hot dogs:

> **140** calories
>
> **3** grams of fat

Two hot dog rolls:
> **220** calories
>
> **3** grams of fat

A grand total of . . . **360** calories and **6** grams of fat. A savings of . . . **240** calories and **31** grams of fat.

It was easier than I thought. It wasn't necessary to live on dry salads with dry tuna. No more suffering through small meals. I promised the scared "Jen" that she would get enough to eat, that she wouldn't starve. Now I was going get the amount of food I needed, while reducing calories and fat.

Regular chunky–style soup (one can):
> **480** calories
>
> **30** grams of fat

Low-fat soup (lots of varieties, one can):
> **260** calories
>
> **3** grams of fat

A savings of . . . **220** calories and **27** grams of fat.

Not all foods are labeled. So, what should you do when you have no way of knowing the fat and calorie content?

If you have no idea what's in a particular food (and your instincts tell you it might be high in fat), assume it to be high in fat, and eat only a little of it.

For example, you're at a party and there's a large dish filled with diced chicken, pasta, with an unidentified sauce. You taste it. It's out of this world! You try to figure out how it's made. ". . . Well, it doesn't seem *too* fatty, but darn is this *good*." There's also a large bowl of fruit salad, and a green salad as well. The best strategy would be to take a *small* scoop of the chicken dish, and load up on the fruit and green salads.

Not having a label to rely on makes choices more difficult, but in a "missing label" situation, use common sense. Don't use the absence of a label as an excuse to give up responsibility. "Oh, there is *no label* on this fettuccini Alfredo, I'm *sure* it's not *that* high in fat." Welcome to the land of denial!

Today, there are many healthy food options on the market. You can find a healthier alternative for just about every fatty food. Most of the time, you'll have more control over choices.

As soon as I started exploring the world of low-fat, healthy foods I was on a roll, filling my cart with the choices I'd discovered. I didn't expect to like all of them, but I was so fed up, so tired of buying size 22 pants, that I was willing to give my new food discoveries a chance.

At the beginning of my successful weight loss, when I was still worried about not getting enough to eat, it was comforting to know that I could still put lots of food in my shopping cart. That felt *good*. I like to see volume and lots of food on my plate. If I had to choose between tiny amounts of fatty, high-calorie foods and realistic portions of low-fat, *sometimes* less flavorful foods, I'd go for volume. For me, that goes back to my fear of *not getting enough*. I could accept a new approach if I knew I *was* going to get enough to eat.

My mother once suggested I have just one small piece of regular cheese. She wondered why I needed to eat a lot of this strange "low-fat and fat-free stuff."

If she only knew! If she only knew how much I wanted to be like her: to forget the ice cream was in the freezer; to slice a small piece of regular cheese, only to wrap up the rest; or to eat just a few greasy potato chips and not go back to the bag again, again, and again until it was empty. She'd never know what it was like to feel overstuffed and guilty. She'd never know what it was like to be me.

My ultimate goal was to learn how to have that one slice of cheese without guilt, without setting myself up for potential disaster. In the meantime—as I was learning to change those behaviors—I saved hundreds of calories a day by switching to low-fat foods.

I learned to love reduced calorie/reduced fat options, particularly the meatless veggie products. It took time, but the results made all the substitutions worth it!

Later, I'll explain how I gradually reintroduced "normal" foods into my diet. I don't want you to think that I live exclusively on low-fat food. I don't. But, during the start-up stage of weight loss, this was the only practical, healthy way to give myself a jump-start.

I still eat many low-fat foods. They allow me the volume of food I need to feel comfortable, but I don't depend on them as much as I did when I began my final, successful weight loss.

When I begin working with weight-loss clients, I show them how many calories and grams of fat they can save by investigating all the different healthy foods on the market. Some get very excited. They leave my office and rush to the grocery store, and in our next session report on all the ways they've found to cut down on fat and calories, while still enjoying lots of food on their plate.

Some clients enthusiastically devote time and energy to experimenting with new foods. They buy low-fat cookbooks and prepare their favorite recipes. "The baked eggplant parmigiana was wonderful, Jennifer! I loved the low-fat cheese sauce and the vegetarian chili!" They launch their weight-loss journey with a positive attitude. I know they will succeed. They're excited, but also prepared to be patient. They're ready to make themselves (not a diet) the priority. For those clients, weight loss is an exciting *challenge.*

"Low-fat" sabotage

Initially, I had lost nearly forty pounds without suffering. I had done it in part by choosing low-fat substitutes for most of the high-fat foods I had eaten in the past. In addition to moving more (I'll explain this later) I had taken the time to create a low-fat version of nearly *all* of my favorite recipes and I'd learned to love them all.

Now, I was a convert. Greasy, oily foods were no longer my first choice. I liked how I felt after eating low-fat meals. I didn't feel bogged down after eating, and eating this way didn't feel like a diet, at least not like any diet *I'd* ever been on. I wasn't hungry! I was eating heartily, while consistently making low-fat choices. And my new way of eating really paid off . . . for a while.

In the beginning, I lost weight because low-fat choices automatically reduced the number of calories I was consuming. But, weight loss isn't just about reducing fat grams. I was about to discover that, the hard way.

After a few months, my weight loss came to a frustrating standstill. I wanted to blame my "dysfunctional metabolism" or my "childhood illness," the story I had *always* relied on to explain my weight problem. But, deep down, I knew the truth. Sure, I had switched to the low-fat versions of all my favorite treats. At first, I was satisfied with a small bag of baked low-fat chips, or a suggested serving of low-fat, frozen yogurt. I amazed myself. But gradually, an old, familiar voice began to whisper, "Jennifer, you're losing weight, you can get away with eating more! It's *low-fat* frozen yogurt; eat a pint. These are *fat-*

free cookies, eat six. You don't *have* to stop at the 'serving size.' This stuff is low fat! *Go for it!"*

Now was the time to reevaluate what I was doing. It was necessary to start recording my calories again. I asked myself, *Which of these low-fat foods am I eating too much of?* I made a list: reduced-fat chips, frozen yogurt, fat-free crackers, fat-free pudding, and fat-free cookies. My commitment to reducing fat in my diet had worked, but I was eating too much low-fat junk! Low-fat foods *still* contain *calories* and, unfortunately, most packaged snack varieties provide little or no nutrition.

After examining my problem, I realized it was time to enter a new phase in my weight loss. Now, I was going to have to choose between eating too many hollow, low-fat calories and my weight goal.

I would have to consider healthier alternatives to the low-fat "void-of-nutrition" choices I was making. It was a painful choice because I was happy with my new low-fat snacks. After all, I'd only recently adjusted to eating lower-fat snacks. Now I was facing another, even more drastic change in my eating, and the part of me that worried about not getting enough food, was scared. But, in spite of my fears, I chose to focus on getting the body I'd always wanted.

I knew what I had to do.

My weight-loss progress finally moved beyond that stalled stage when I began to replace empty, fat-free products (low-fiber, high-sugar foods) with fruits, vegetables, and whole grain products.

Every eating opportunity now provided nutrition. For the first time in my life, *I fueled my body. I didn't just fill it.*

As often as I could (I didn't ask myself to be perfect) I replaced a snack, such as six fat-free cookies, with another choice—a small serving of high fiber cereal or yogurt mixed with a handful of cereal, or cottage cheese with a serving of whole wheat crackers. Fresh fruit accompanied my sandwich instead of baked potato chips. Often, I snacked on yogurt and fruit instead of fat-free cookies. My focus became nutrition and good health, not just weight loss.

To my surprise, I was more satisfied with meals that included healthy food choices.

I'm convinced that one important reason we keep going back to the box, back to the bag, back to the container, is because our bodies are looking for something more in the way of nutrition and we don't get it from these packaged snack foods! That may be why I have *never* met a client who consistently overeats *healthy* foods. How often do we binge on yogurt, fresh fruit, high-fiber/low-sugar cereal, or chopped veggies?

"Jennifer, I don't know what happened! I opened a bag of carrots and that was that. The next thing I knew the whole bag was gone! So, since I already felt guilty, I decided to binge on the plums!" Ever heard *that* one? Me neither!

To be honest, this nutrition-targeting behavior change was not easy. Healthy eating takes *planning*. Grabbing a package of fat-free crackers as I ran out the door was *easy*. I could munch them on the go. When I was ravenous, I loved being able to tear into a bag of low-fat chips. A commitment to better health, *not just* weight loss, was going to require that I *think*. I'd have to prepare. That's something that those of us who have food issues, hate to do. When we're really hungry, we don't want to take extra time *before* eating.

Fast food is very popular in this country. Unfortunately, it isn't just convenient; it's also mostly high in fat and calories. Most dieters already know that. But, low-fat food can also be fast and easy—*too* easy. And that's how it still gets us overeaters into trouble. Too much of even a good thing is still too much.

Crave the taste of potato chips? Pining for a dish of ice cream? Do you *have* to have a muffin with your coffee? Fat-free or low-fat versions of these foods are always the better weight-loss choice. They'll save you many calories and (obviously) lots of fat. **But, these products are useful *only* if you can stop at one serving.** If you use them as anything but a stand-in for the high-fat, high-calorie versions of the same foods, you'll find yourself in big trouble. It's so easy to slide into an it's-low-fat—I'll-eat-the-bag mentality. Ultimately, that results in a big increase in our calorie consumption, and, because we're feeling safe, because of that low-fat label, it sneaks up on us. Be careful not to abuse these products.

Give Me Five

Eat five times a day? How could that work? On a diet you try to eat less, right? *Wrong*! You're not dieting anymore, remember?

When people are trying to lose weight, they generally try to watch what they eat, or eat very little, during the first two-thirds of their day. In general, the average overweight person eats only about one-third of his or her calories *before* 3:00 p.m., and the other two-thirds *after* 3:00 P.M.

We dieters are most motivated to eat less early in the day. It's easy for us to eat a light breakfast. I have yet to meet a client who eats a greasy, fast food breakfast on a regular basis. We often ignore our nutrition needs during the day. We have other things to focus on. Then the day starts winding down. Winding down puts us in danger.

For many people with weight issues, time on their hands results in mindless eating. At the end of the day we reward ourselves with food, we pamper ourselves with food, we console ourselves with food, we soothe ourselves with food, we comfort ourselves with food. Whatever our reasons, the result is the same, we overeat. Then, we often feel guilty, angry, and miserable. These negative feelings only add to our problem—we don't feel good about ourselves, which leads to more self-destructive food behavior.

Clients often react with fear when I suggest fueling their bodies regularly during the day. That's because ten out of ten of them list their problem eating time as after 3:00 P.M. "Jennifer, I don't want to add *more* calories during the day. I'll gain weight! I already eat much too much food. I don't want to add to those calories! I can't control myself late in the day."

There are exceptions to the rule, but most people wait until they get home to do their most destructive eating because, in their home, structure and restrictions are eliminated. That's where we can eat as much as we want, in private.

Until clients and I develop an eating plan that works for them, I ask them to keep a daily food log, so we can chart their problem-eating patterns. When I examine these logs, I often see familiar behaviors. Though there are exceptions, most clients (even those who are very overweight) manage to restrict their eating in the morning. Breakfast is often something as harmless as toast, a bagel, cereal, a small muffin, or (worst yet) nothing at all. Many of my clients bring a light lunch to work or order out. Most people don't engage in serious, destructive behavior until their day winds down.

Interestingly, if fatty foods or junky foods *are* eaten early in the day, eating behaviors often become even *more* destructive in the evening. That's because we develop the what-the-hell-I've-already-blown-it attitude. There are exceptions to this late-in-the-day eating, but it usually isn't until my clients are in familiar territory, at home at the end of the day, or in a relaxed setting, that they completely lose control.

I've observed that overeating at night is often the result of poor nutrition during the day. The end-of-day eater probably hasn't met their nutritional needs. I believe that when people crave certain foods, they may actually need nourishment. Unfortunately, we often respond to our body's cry for nutrients by giving it more hollow calories. It becomes a vicious cycle. We *fill* our bodies; we don't *fuel* our bodies. We stuff our bodies; we don't feed our bodies.

Here's a strange phenomenon: we people with food issues are *very* resistant to the suggestion that we should get plenty to eat. We cycle-dieters are familiar with deprivation. We're prepared to struggle to control our eating. But, when I suggest that they eat every few hours, clients look confused. "I'll *gain* weight Jennifer! I can't lose weight on this much food!"

But, what has deprivation eating done for them in the past? We all know the results that "starvation" diets—in fact, *all* diets—produce.

Think of an imbalanced-eating day as a "mini-diet." We have control in the morning, just like the beginning stage of a diet. As the day goes on, control diminishes, just like that decline stage of a diet. Next thing we know, it's the end of the day, we're home and we're tired of being deprived. We eat a little of this, a little more of that; before the evening is over, we may have stuffed ourselves. That sounds exactly like all my diet-focused, weight-loss attempts. And that's exactly how they used to end. I'd give up and give in to every temptation I had denied myself, because I was fed up with being underfed.

To clients who put themselves on daily mini-diets, my recommendation that they eat in a more balanced way sounds like giving up on weight loss. It's so hard for us to de-program a life of diet brainwashing. How can my suggestion they eat five mini-meals a day result in anything but weight gain? They assume they'll continue to eat just as much at night.

The lure of strict control, through gimmicky diets, is so strong we'll repeatedly go back to it, rather than try something that sounds painless.

When clients increase what they eat throughout the day, by planning *balanced, nutrition-focused meals and snacks,* late-in-the-day eating decreases.

Some Examples:

Breakfast: A healthy, hearty, balanced meal such as half of a whole-grain bagel with low-fat cream cheese and a piece of fruit, or a bowl of high-fiber cereal topped with fruit.

Snack: Between 9:00–11:00 A.M. Something healthy and satisfying before lunch: yogurt, crackers with cottage cheese, or fruit, for example, a banana with a *small* amount of peanut butter.

Lunch: Lunch should be the biggest meal of the day. I use this meal as an opportunity to give myself high-quality nutrition, such as a veggie burger, a salad with grilled shrimp or chicken, or a sandwich of hummus and vegetables. My goal is to avoid feeling "starved" by dinnertime.

Snack: Between 3:00–5:00 p.m., I eat something light but nourishing—another yogurt, a few pieces of fruit, a bowl of soup, or a few crackers with a small amount of cheese.

Dinner: When my eating day has been nutritious, I'm in control. **This is the key:** Don't let yourself get frantically hungry! I'm generally able to keep my dinner portions under control—a modest serving of fish with veggies and a salad, or a lean burger with a baked potato topped with low-fat cheese, salsa, and a salad.

Eating this way has provided me with the discipline and control I've always wanted. Now, I'm able to approach a meal like a *lean* person does. I no longer feel that frantic sense of "starvation." Being calm allows me to take that extra time needed to plan a healthy, balanced meal.

Five mini-meals a day is important for us, because of our broken hunger meter. It's the same as a broken gas gauge. If the car you drove all day had no reliable way to measure how much fuel it had, you'd *have* to fill it up regularly. If you gave it fuel several times throughout the day, you'd never have to worry about running out of gas.

Focus on *fueling* your body throughout the day. Never go for more than a few hours without a little healthy snack.

Within two years after I became "fit," I took a job at a local YMCA, teaching weight management.

Since I had a reputation at the gym as the weight-loss coach, people often paid attention to what I ate. One day, I walked by two women who were working at the front desk. I was eating a sandwich I had brought from home that contained veggies, hummus, and low-fat cheese.

The women at the desk called me over. "So, what gives, Jennifer? All you ever do is eat! Every time you walk by us, you're eating something! How come you're not gaining weight?"

I understood how I must have looked to them. They had a valid point. By dieting standards, I *was* always eating.

"Have you ever paid attention to *what* I'm eating?" I asked. "It's either yogurt, fruit, a healthy, low-fat sandwich, or cut up veggies." I was aware that in the evening, they often ordered a large pizza, or frantically made a "meal" from the vending machines even though they were struggling with weight issues. They ate so little during the day, that by the end of the day, they were starving.

Yes, I was eating all day, but not just to eat. I was providing my body with nutrition and great, satisfying fuel. They were eating less often than I was, true. But *what* were they eating? Hollow calories, lots of fat, and junk, and most of it late in the day. At the end of the day, their bodies were still calling for nutrition.

When am I most dangerous around food? (Yes, I'm *still* dangerous around food.) When do I let go of all the healthy behaviors I've worked so hard to make a part of my life?

Answer: When I've gone too long without food. To this day, I will eat three times what I need when I enter a meal "starving." Remember the hunger meter? We know "starving," we know "stuffed." We must focus on staying in the in-between gray area. Never starve; never stuff.

As a child, I remember experiencing frantic, food-related feelings. Sometimes, when Mom picked me up from school, I would beg her to drive me to McDonald's because I was "starving." We'd arrive at the drive-thru and I'd want two of everything. "Mom, I want two cheeseburgers, two fries, and a huge Coke." What she said next was maddening. "Jennifer, I'll get you *one* cheeseburger and if, in twenty minutes, you're *still* hungry, I'll drive back to get you more."

I can trace my first experience with feeling fury around this time. How could she do this? Here I was a young, starving child and she wouldn't buy everything I wanted to eat. It made me want to cry. She didn't understand. It wasn't until twenty years later that I began to understand what she had been *trying* to do.

She knew better. She knew that my announcement that I was "starving" didn't mean I should double my food intake. (Remember those two shrimp left on her plate?)

She was right about the amounts. I'd eat the single cheeseburger and in less than half an hour forget that I'd originally asked for more.

Whenever we go into a meal feeling as though we are "starving" we're convinced there is no way our hunger can be satisfied by a *normal* serving of anything. We're running on "empty" and it feels bottomless.

Don't allow yourself to get into a "starvation" mode. Staying ahead of your hunger will help you find a healthy way to approach weight loss. If you regularly eat hearty, healthy mini-meals throughout the day, your destructive, self-sabotaging eating habits will be brought under control.

Light My Fire

We've talked about "when," now let's talk about "what" and "why."

To describe the way our bodies use the fuel we provide, the best analogy I can think of is the "fireplace." In my analogy, logs represent food—nutritious and non-nutritious.

Fireplace #1: This fireplace has a few gray coals and one red coal, but no genuine flames. The people who maintain this fireplace are never consistent. They have a history of on-again/off-again dieting and exercise. They may follow a weight-reduction program enthusiastically, for a short time, but eventually they always give up and go back to their former, weight-gaining lifestyle.

When you visualize this fireplace, imagine what happens when its owner suddenly dumps a load of soggy, slow- or non-burning logs, right on top of those few, fragile coals. That single red coal not only isn't fueled, it's nearly snuffed out. If the logs burn at all, they just lay, smoldering, in that fireplace, until the next, heavy, soggy load of fuel is thrown on top of them.

The wet, soggy logs represent fatty, low-nutrition foods eaten in large amounts. That's why this person's fireplace *never* burns efficiently. On average, this fireplace owner is at least forty pounds overweight.

Fireplace #2: These people maintain a fireplace that has a few red coals, and a few, small flickering flames. They may have stayed faithful to moderate exercise throughout their life. They eat in a "mostly" healthy way, but they eat too much, too often. They try to diet, now and then, and they get some exercise. They may walk two to three times a week or they may engage in some other activity that requires "movement." Some of their fuel burns efficiently, but not all of it. On average, these people are about fifteen to forty pounds overweight.

Fireplace #3: These people maintain a bonfire! They *need* a steady supply of fuel. They exercise vigorously four or more times a week. They're very active, never sedentary for long. Generally, they eat nutritious food. These fireplace owners are rarely overweight. After all, you can toss the occasional "soggy logs" (three pieces of pizza, for example) into a fire like *this* one, and it will *still* burn. Physical activity keeps their fuel-burning efficiency, at a high level.

Until I lost weight for the last, successful time, I was a fireplace #1. I moved very little, and stuffed my fireplace with high-fat, low-nutrition fuel. I ate the most after 3:00 P.M. until bedtime. I not only buried my *one* red coal with soggy logs. I allowed those weight-producing logs to smolder through the night.

My typical day began with a skipped breakfast or a tiny one, on the run. Often, lunch was a large sub-like sandwich. It had to be filling and quick, because, by then, I was starving. In the evening, I'd eat a big, easy unplanned dinner, something sweet for dessert, usually followed by late night snacks. (Did I fail to mention, there were also countless, mindless treats in between?)

By not eating breakfast, or eating a tiny breakfast, my *one and only red coal* started the day "fuel deprived." I'd crave food because I had nothing of quality to burn during the morning. Not understanding how important it was to eat in a balanced way, I'd often go hours between meals. I'd reach "starvation-level" hunger, and *now* I was old enough to drive *myself* to the drive-thru. I no longer had my mom telling me to buy half of what I thought I needed. I was a girl on a mission!

My single coal burned what it could (which wasn't much) and the rest of what I ate was stored primarily as fat.

And I wondered why I was over seventy pounds overweight.

And yet, I was famous for complaining! "I don't eat *that* much, and look at me! My metabolism is terrible!"

Because I *believed* I had a faulty metabolism, I was easily discouraged. There were days when I woke up with a "who cares" mindset. "I don't really care about my weight. I'll eat whatever I choose, whatever and whenever I want it. Who really gives a damn?" I refer to those days as "burnout" days—tired of thinking about which foods were good or bad. If there was cold, leftover pizza on the counter, I ate it. If there was a box of doughnuts in the house, I'd start my day with a few of those. Then, because I started the day with bad foods, the rest of the day didn't matter. I would continue to eat foods that I typically considered off limits. By keeping myself fuel-deprived, just stuffed all day long, you can imagine what I was doing to my fireplace!

But eventually, I began to examine my behaviors. I compared them to the behaviors of people I thought looked really good.

One of my biggest problems was that I hated exercise. It was obvious to me that the people I knew who looked fit *moved*. I didn't, I had little energy. The idea of exercising, the very thought of it, made me tired. It was overwhelming. Although I hadn't yet figured it out, I had no energy because I wasn't giving my body any high energy fuel such as healthy foods in moderate amounts. Also, I was carrying around a load of fat that was the equivalent of a seventy-pound backpack. None of these active lean types were carrying any excess baggage. But, I assumed, because I was so tired all the time, there was something wrong with me.

Fruits, vegetables, high-fiber foods, whole-grains, low-fat proteins are high-quality, good nutrition, efficiently burning logs. The condition of your fireplace—and your energy level—depends on the type of fuel *you* provide.

When I was overweight, I consumed approximately 2,500 or more calories a day (almost *all* of them junky, poor nutrition calories). My clothing size stayed between 18 and 22.

Today, I can easily maintain my weight loss and consume around 2,000 calories a day, but almost all of them are highly nutritional, as well as satisfying.

Occasionally I splurge and eat four slices of pizza, with a serving of french fries, and an ice cream sundae. But, I now know if I exercise on a consistent basis, I can maintain a bonfire. I can get away with the occasional caloriefest.

In my dieting past I never thought about changing my fireplace; I always focused on fuel deprivation. My new approach to weight loss succeeded because I dedicated myself to eating differently while gradually changing the way my body burned the fuel I provided.

I also became conscious of how I *talked* about food.

Things I *never* heard my healthy, "in-shape" friends say:

- "I feel gross; I ate too much."
- "I shouldn't have eaten french fries. They're 'bad.' I might as well eat junk for the rest of the day!"
- "I don't have time to exercise."
- "I'm not hungry, but I'm going to eat anyhow."
- "I need to lose weight. I'll start Monday."

My old, self-defeating phrases were being replaced by my positive, I-can-do-it mentality. I *could* develop a realistic, satisfying, eating plan while achieving my weight-loss goal.

I did.

In time, my hot coals became flames.

Social Survival

Social situations provided foods that gave me an opportunity to go wild, and I often did. So, I always began a diet prepared to miss out on social events. Having no control over the food being served made me panic. Amounts were often unlimited. Choices were usually high fat. It was like walking through a minefield. Telling myself I couldn't eat rarely worked. Putting unrealistic restrictions on myself, often caused me to eat twice as much. But, if I didn't eat at all, I might have to explain myself to the hostess and other guests.

Remember when you were a little kid and your mom said, "Don't eat that before dinner, it will spoil your appetite?" Well, now it's time to spoil your appetite!

Some friends and I were invited to a cookout. The hostess, Terry, was famous for her fatty foods and incredible dips. At the time, I was about halfway to my weight-loss goal.

The thought of spending a day at this woman's house terrified me. Delicious high-fat foods *everywhere*—for five hours! It was a food disaster in the making.

I decided to approach the event in a new way. Before heading to the cookout, I poured myself a *large* bowl of high-fiber cereal, loaded with fruit. By the time I finished the cereal, I was stuffed!

"What are you doing?" my girlfriend asked. "Are you crazy? We're on our way to Terry's, and she'll have plenty of food!"

"Exactly, and I don't want to be starving when we get there," I explained.

When we arrived at the cookout, it was just what I expected: cheesy artichoke dips, fatty cold cuts, luscious desserts, and creamy casseroles. The high-fat choices went on and on. But because of the cereal and fruit, I was "okay." In control. Calm.

I walked around and surveyed the selections and found a huge fruit salad. *Yippee!* I thought. *I can eat this, and it won't undermine my weight loss.* Normally I would have eaten at least six pieces of Terry's famous cheesy garlic bread and then (feeling the "two G's," *gross* and *guilty*), I would have continued to stuff myself with other things all night. Instead, I ate some fruit salad, two pieces of garlic bread and stopped.

I have frightening memories of the days before I learned to handle social situations, when I *didn't* stay ahead of my hunger.

I remember one party in particular. At the time, I was down a few sizes and felt on top of the world. "I can handle *any* food situation," I told myself. "I'm a new person."

It was a tenth birthday party for a dog, and we were invited to bring our pet. I knew the hostess was serving doggie biscuits and beef jerky. Not *my* favorites. It sounded like a safe food environment.

I couldn't have been more wrong! Sure, there were "doggie goodies," but there was also a big assortment of "human" treats, too. Guests had not only brought their dogs, but cookies, cakes, cheesy spreads, chips, and potato salad. My dog was in heaven, and so was I. To make things worse, I arrived "*starving.*"

"I'll just have a little of this and a smidgen of that," I promised myself, as I fixed myself a small plate.

But after eating some of the offerings, my negative voice soon took over. "Now you've blown it, Jennifer. You shouldn't have eaten *any* of this stuff! Your day is ruined! Oh . . . and by the way, those cookies, right over there, they have your name on them."

In those still-learning days, I only gave myself two choices: completely in control (perfect) or completely out of control (destructive).

I can still remember the drive home from that party. It was just me and my dog. Sure, she ate her share of treats, but she didn't feel like I did—stuffed and miserable. She seemed to stare at me, in a judgmental way, like she was thinking, "Why'd ya do that?" (Or was it just my guilty conscience?) The point is, I learned my lesson. I couldn't just *tell* myself I'd be fine. I had to eat before any food-related event.

There's a basic difference between trim, average eaters and us. After eating a hearty portion of something before going to a party, someone with no food issues simply wouldn't eat any more. They'd say something ridiculous like, "Boy, that creamy artichoke dip looks delicious, but I'm just not hungry."

We who struggle with weight problems often eat for *taste*. Taste continues to tempt and delight us even though we're not hungry. We don't equate "not hungry" with "satisfied." As long as it still tastes wonderful, we'll continue to eat it.

That's why eating *before* we go to a social event won't *always* solve our overeating problem, but it *will* help, on average, about 85 percent of the time. So that means if you stick with this strategy you'll only derail about 15 percent of the time. That's good enough to keep you on track, as you head toward your weight-loss goal.

At Terry's cookout, when I chose to eat beforehand, I wasn't as gratified as I might have been if I'd stuffed myself with her fatty treats. Honestly, I baited myself. "Why not go for it, Jennifer? This is a once-a-year event!"

Being a "fatty food" bystander—a nonparticipant in this "foodfest"—wasn't as much fun. But "fun" wasn't the issue. I had to choose between doing what I had *always* done—stuffing myself, like someone in an all-you-can-eat eating contest—or staying focused on my most important priority; my life-changing weight-loss goal. I had made the best choice. I left Terry's once-a-year cookout feeling proud of myself.

Later, when I arrived home after Terry's party, I felt a sense of accomplishment. I knew I had taken a major step toward achieving my weight-loss goal.

After my success at Terry's cookout, I tried my eat-beforehand strategy again. My best friend asked me to lunch. She wanted to go to a specific restaurant, but I knew it offered few healthy choices. Normally, I would have asked to go to another place, but this one was close for both of us and I didn't want to be a pain. So, instead, I made a quick stop at home. There, I opened a can of vegetable soup, heated it in the microwave, and drank it on the road. (Yes, I did have bits of the soup stuck to my face when I arrived to meet my friend. You try drinking soup, from a wide-mouthed container, while you're driving! But, I had accomplished what I wanted to do.) The point is I arrived with my appetite under control. This control gave me the ability to make smarter choices. I was able to select one of the few healthy items on the menu: a garden salad, with shrimp, without taking her up on her offer to share her nacho appetizer. (My friend had arrived "starving.")

In theory, I shouldn't have wanted to eat at all, since I arrived at these two social situations already having eaten. But that's not how I operate. What this strategy provides is the control that makes it possible to make healthier food choices. I *still* ate at those events; I just didn't eat in a destructive, self-sabotaging way.

Eight years later, I still use this approach.

Here are a few hearty pre-social event snack suggestions:

- Half bagel with a small serving of peanut butter
- A few small pieces of cheese and a piece of fruit
- One bowl of high-fiber cereal with fruit
- One handful of nuts with a few pieces of fruit
- One banana with a small serving of peanut butter
- A large yogurt with high-fiber cereal mixed in

- A serving of high-fiber crackers with a serving of hummus
- Half a tuna sandwich, with whole grain bread and light mayo, loaded up with lettuce and tomato
- Half a turkey sandwich with light mayo, lettuce and tomato
- Oatmeal with fruit

I Can't Stop

There are some people who have no problem eating small portions of any food that they love. But, unfortunately, I belong to that bigger group. My group knows that at times just a taste of any food they truly love will send them into a downward spiral of out-of-control eating.

I have a "danger foods" list. Even though I've maintained my weight loss for eight years, there are still foods that I'm unable to eat in a reasonable and healthy way. It begins with a harmless first taste and usually ends only when the box, carton, bag, or container is completely empty.

I'll share my "I can't stop" list:

- Malted milk balls—So light and airy—twenty, thirty, who's counting?
- Ginger snaps—They must put some secret ingredient in these cookies! I'm an addict!
- Cheese (displayed on a buffet table)—Do I have to explain?
- Chocolate chip cookies—Slice and bake (if there's any dough left for actual cookies)!
- Cheese curls—Note: because of their unnatural, neon-orange color, we were not allowed to have these as children. I have since made up for lost time.
- Coffee cake—My all-time favorite!
- Ice cream—Oooo la la! I can have one scoop. Not!

There are more, but why embarrass myself further? The sad truth? I'm a high-fat food lover. Even today, when these foods are in front of me, I feel nervous, insecure. Can I, will I, stop? History proves I can't. I usually eat them until I can't eat any more. I eat them in large amounts, expecting to make myself temporarily sick of them. "If I *stuff* myself maybe I won't crave this taste for awhile!" Because I don't want to sabotage myself, I generally keep these foods out of my house.

Notice that my out-of-control list doesn't include any healthy, natural foods like fruits or vegetables? No whole-grain products. No yogurt. Can you imagine being at a party and hearing someone say, "Please move that bowl of vegetables out of my reach. I'm out of control. I can't stop eating them"? If that were the case, none of us would have a weight problem.

During my weight loss, I sometimes bought ginger snaps. I'd tell myself I *could* eat only the number the label said was a serving size—three. I would leave the store fixated on those cookies. I *wanted* them. As soon as I got in my car, I removed three from the box, then put the box out of range in the back seat, in a location nearly impossible to reach. After I devoured my "allowed" three, in less than a minute, the cookies began to call from the back of my car, *"Jennifer, we taste sooo good. We're fat-free, too. Eat more of us. It won't matter . . . !"*

At the first red light, I attempted to get to the cookies. I contorted my body into a position I didn't think was possible. I must have looked like Gumby! But I couldn't reach them! What did I have that was long, thin, and hooked and would extend my reach? I spotted it, the perfect tool: my antitheft, steering wheel bar! Frantic, I used the bar to slide the cookie box closer.

You'd think I was someone thrown overboard. I was as desperate as a person trying to reach a lifeboat! Getting to those cookies was like a life or death proposition.

Serving size? Who cared about serving size? I ate four . . . eight . . . ten . . . until, at last, I was all crunched out. Ugh. *I won't be buying them for awhile. I feel gross.*

I'd done it again. Yet, after every one of these episodes I told myself, "Next time I buy these cookies, I'll be able to keep myself under control. I couldn't tell myself *never* to buy cookies again. Ginger snaps were one of my favorite foods. The thought of "never" was too painful. So I *had* to convince myself that next time I could maintain control, even if I couldn't. It was only after about twenty broken promises that I decided I couldn't buy them anymore.

But the belief that some of my favorite foods had to be kept completely out of my life worried me. Would I *ever* be able to live in a normal way around my trigger foods? I had my doubts.

Sometime after that, a friend and I went to a department store, where, lo and behold, the Easter candy was on sale. Easter had come and gone so all the candy was half price. Malted milk Easter eggs happen to be on my I-can't-stop list.

"I'm buying these," I said. "I'll just eat a few."

Lie number one: I've never eaten a "few" malted milk balls in my life! When I eat them, I eat them until I'm nearly sick.

"Do *you* want some? I can't eat all these by myself." Lie number two. Who was I trying to kid? I could eat *two* containers all by myself. My poor friend actually asked for a couple. I shot her a look that said, "Ask for another one and you're dead!"

I began to stuff them in my mouth while we were still walking through the store. Three . . . eight . . . ten . . . twelve! I was starting to feel gross. Fifteen . . . twenty . . . then they were all gone. I'd eaten them all, before we left the store! Now I felt stuffed, guilty, and miserable. How familiar!

The biggest lie was lie number three: "I won't be eating malted milk balls again for at least ten years!"

Why does this happen with some foods and not others? If I had purchased another half-price candy like jelly beans, or milk-chocolate eggs, I might still *want* to eat the entire container, but I *could* stop.

But certain foods will always trigger something that sends me on a destructive, downward spiral. Is it the taste, the texture, the satisfaction they provide? I wish I knew . . .

I have a possible answer, though it's not scientific. It's based on what I've observed. I believe our bodies sometimes call for more nutrition, but we respond to that call by overeating high-fat and/or sugar-loaded foods.

How often do we lose control on nutrition-packed foods such as vegetables, fruits, beans, whole-grain, high-fiber cereals, and whole-grain breads? How often do we lose control while eating lean protein such as fish, skinless chicken breast, or turkey? When was the last time you said, "I can't stop eating these green beans, and this fruit salad! Please, take it away!" We never binge on the foods that provide us with the most nutrition. When we eat those foods we're giving our bodies what they *need*. Our body doesn't *have* to say, "You're going to have to eat a ton of that junk, in order to provide me with any nutrition *at all!*"

I use the following "step" analogy to explain my nutrition theory to clients. For example, an ear of corn. Consider the number of steps it takes to process fresh corn into a cheese-puff snack. That snack certainly doesn't *look* like the original, nutritious vegetable. By the time the corn reaches its new form, it's so far from its original state that most of its nutritional value is gone. Nearly all of the vitamins, minerals, and fiber have been stripped! We eat serving after serving of the processed product not realizing our body is being seduced by taste while desperately searching for nutritional satisfaction. "Well, I didn't get any nutrition from *that* serving, I'll have another . . . and another." Soon the hollow snack is gone and we're still nutritionally deprived.

For me, eating a baked potato is satisfying. I rarely want more than one. But ask me about potato chips. If I open a bag, I'm on a munching mission. The fat, salt, and sugar added to most of these processed foods, greatly expands the flavor—most people would argue for the better. These flavors, which are designed to quickly target our most receptive taste buds, certainly contribute to our lack of control. But I believe the absence of nutrition in these products plays more of a role than we realize.

Bran cereal with raisins has a sweet taste, and one bowl is usually satisfying. But, give me a nutritionally empty, sugar cereal, and I'll attack the box, eating until it's gone. The bran cereal has retained most of its fiber, vitamins, and minerals. The process that turns whole wheat into bran cereal doesn't involve many steps. The trip from wheat to light and puffy sugar cereal—not counting the cute cartoon on the box—involves several, nutrition-stripping steps. That's why, though we're stuffed, we're often still unsatisfied.

Do you have an I-can't-stop foods list, foods that once you taste them are nearly impossible to put away? Do you ever dip into a bag, box, or container of something again and again, unable to resist the taste, eating until it is gone? If you had to guess, how many steps would you say your I-can't-stop foods are from their original form?

List your I-can't-stop foods. Circle the ones you consistently make available. Can't accept the fact that you should never have them? Me, too. But try using the following tips.

1. Don't kid yourself.

We repeatedly make the same, unrealistic promise to ourselves: "I'll just have one serving, maybe two, three max." But the truth is we almost never stop until we overeat our trigger foods.

Be honest. Ask yourself, "Is making this particular food available to me asking for trouble?" If you answer "yes," then get it out of your life. I know, I know, it's unrealistic to say you'll *never* have that trigger food again, but don't make it *easy* to get your hands on it.

2. Don't linger or hover.

Today, if I find myself near a candy dish, filled (for example) with malted milk balls, I don't take a handful and then hover around the candy dish. I know better.

If I'm at a party and there's a cheese and cracker platter, I keep some distance between that platter and me. If I don't, I'm begging for disaster.

If I can't bear to leave without having at least a small taste, I'll wait until I'm ready to leave, then, I'll take a tiny amount with me for the ride home. I've learned to allow myself the taste of a trigger food only when I can avoid exposing myself to the danger of overeating them.

I have my car serviced at a shop where the owners provide mini coffee cakes in the waiting room. Once, when repairs took an hour, I took one, two, three coffee cakes. *Is anyone looking?* Six. Ugggh— stuffed! The next time, I controlled myself because I took only one, *on my way out the door.* I allowed myself the taste, and avoided the weight-loss sabotage.

I no longer buy ice cream to take home. Instead, I go to the local stand, order a serving, and drive away.

How I wish I could eat like my mom or anyone one else who is free of food issues. "Oh, I forgot about this pesky ice cream. Now it's all freezer burned." One little slice of cheese, and Mom's had enough. She might—heaven forbid—spoil her appetite before dinner!

Realistically, I can only hope that as my years of weight maintenance continue, more of my food behaviors will change. *Many already have.* In the meantime, I have to remind myself regularly, that some foods can *still* set me up for disaster, but fortunately, as time goes on, my list is getting smaller. Today, I can actually eat a small serving of many of my former trigger foods and stop in time, before I do damage. What a powerful and satisfying feeling that gives me!

I don't believe in making *any* foods off limits. We have to learn to live with them, because rigid, unrealistic rules will only come back to haunt us.

Besides, I love those I-can't-stop foods and they tend to make pop-up appearances.

Who knows? In a few years I might be able to make a malted milk flavored coffee cake, with ice cream, topped with crumbled cheese curls and eat one piece and push it away. Until then, I pick and choose my food carefully.

4

The Safety of Routine

The Importance of Stocking Up

I've been able to maintain a seventy-pound weight loss for more than eight years because I changed my eating behaviors. One of my strategies requires that I *never* miss my weekly trip to the grocery store. I always have healthy choices available to me.

I learned the hard way that a weekly "stock-up" trip is critical to weight loss.

At the time I began my seventy-pound weight loss, I had three roommates and lived in a house *filled* with junk food.

At that time I was working a twenty-hour week, and attending college. I'd often come home starved, but as part of my new-habits approach to weight loss, I had promised myself I would never begin a meal in starvation mode. Because of my hectic schedule, sticking to my new eat-five-times-a-day rule was very challenging.

I'd come home and rummage through the fridge, searching frantically for *anything* I could eat that wouldn't lead to disaster. Because I wasn't yet shopping regularly, and was usually out of healthy selections, I'd feel frustrated. Choices were limited and high fat. My roommates and I had a what's-mine-is-yours policy. Even if you didn't buy it, you could eat whatever you wanted, as long as you replaced it.

Oh, I'd say to myself, *I'm out of low-fat cheese, so I'll eat a little of Cathy's regular cheese, just a piece or two or three or four. ...*

Eating my roommates' high-fat food was a poor choice. I'd quickly lose control. My sabotaging "voice" would take over. *Jennifer, you shouldn't have eaten all that cheese. You've blown it. Today is wrecked! You might as well finish the package.*

That voice always won. I can't count the number of times I apologized to Cathy for eating all her crackers, cheese, candy, ice cream, etc. Cathy was one of *those* people who didn't even know her food items were missing, which made eating them even easier. I guess that's why Cathy didn't have a weight problem.

Oh, how I wanted to be like Cathy! If one of my roomies ate so much as a tablespoon of *my* frozen yogurt, I'd notice. I'd be in a state of panic until it was replaced.

Eventually, I realized that unless I faithfully provided myself with a supply of healthy food choices, I was going to completely undermine my weight-loss success. To reach my goal, I *had* to keep my supply of healthy food choices well stocked.

I studied my schedule to find shopping opportunities. Monday was out of the question; I had four morning classes and I had to be at work by 3:00 P.M. Tuesdays were out as well, same problem as Monday. Wednesdays were a possibility, because I had a two-hour block of free time in the late afternoon. However, the store was always very busy at that hour. I don't like busy grocery stores. I'd save Wednesday as a backup day. Forget Thursday—that was a double-shift day at work. By process of elimination, I decided to designate Sunday morning for shopping. I could be at the store when it opened, and get in and out quickly. Sunday it was!

Eight years later, I'm still faithful to that shopping schedule and I've *never* run out of healthy selections.

Maintaining a supply of healthy food choices was critical to my weight-loss success, but I assumed it was just important to *me*. That was before I began weight-loss coaching. I soon realized that running out of healthy choices also produces disastrous results for my clients. It's the make-or-break weight-loss issue.

Client: "Jennifer, I had a crazy week. I had to bring the kids to soccer, football, and hockey! I never got a chance to grocery shop. We ate a lot of take-out this week, and I've been eating on the run. It wasn't a progress week. I'm sure I didn't lose weight."

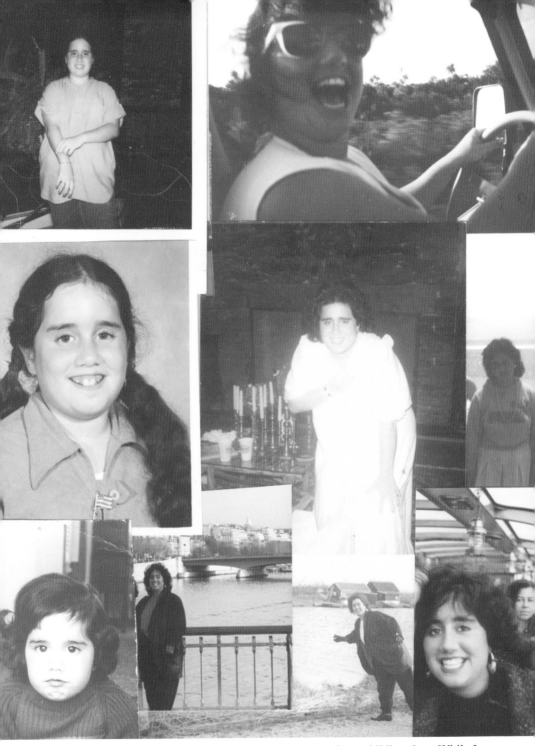

My "before" photos capture various stages of weight gain from childhood on. While I sometimes managed to take some weight off, until I changed my approach to weight loss, I always gained it back. I was always the life of every party and the class clown.

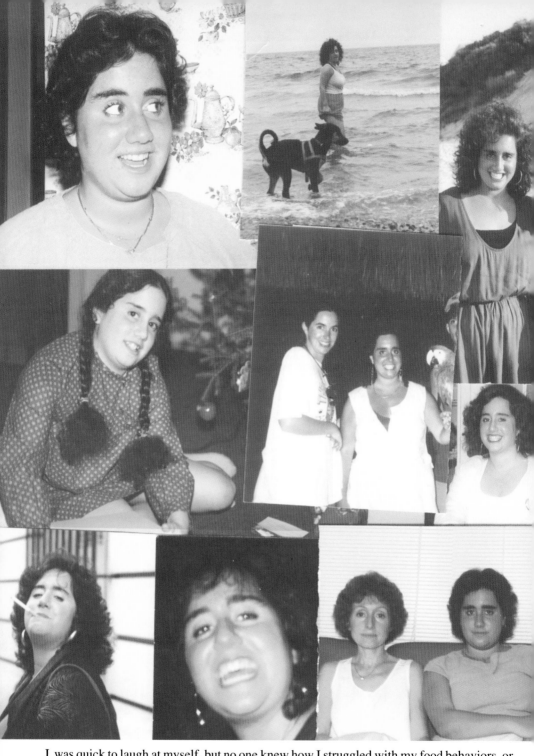

I was quick to laugh at myself, but no one knew how I struggled with my food behaviors, or how I longed to have a body I could be comfortable in and be proud of. My mom (next to me, lower right) always managed to leave the last little shrimp on her plate.

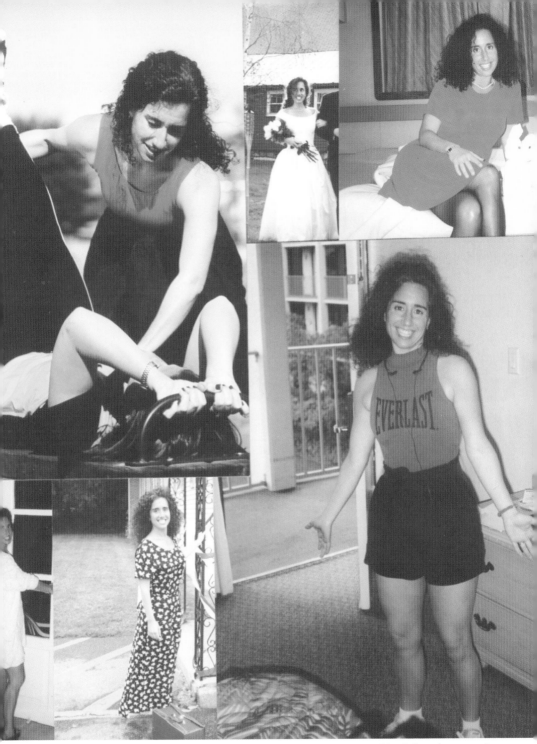

Achieving permanent weight-loss success completely changed my life. I found energy I never dreamed I had. Because dieting was no longer my focus, I now had time for countless other things, as these "after" photos show.

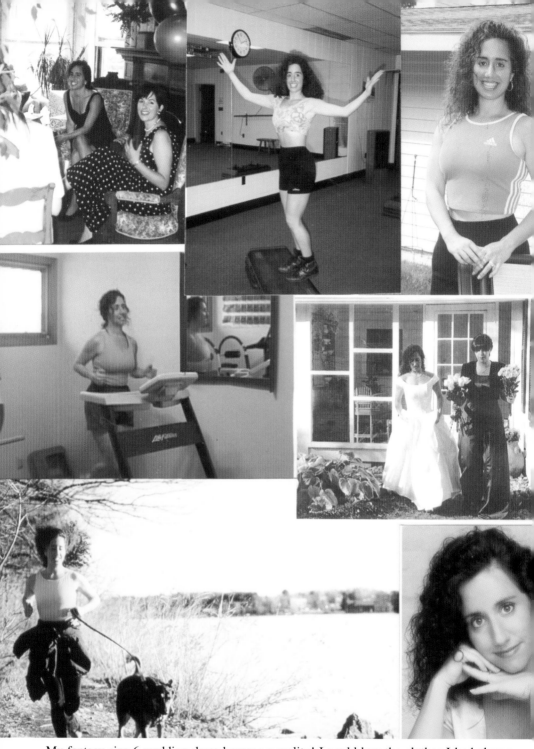

My fantasy size 6 wedding dress became a reality! I could buy the clothes I had always longed to wear. It is easier to smile when you know you will never face another diet. I no longer suffer or struggle to stay thin, yet I have maintained my seventy-pound weight loss.

This client's problem is common. After checking her food chart, I asked why she ate four slices of pizza. "I came home starving, Jennifer. My husband had ordered pizza. I ate pizza because there was *nothing* else in the house. I ate four pieces before I could stop myself!"

This is exactly what you don't want to happen.

Making a list of your favorite healthy options and *never* running out of them is part of your commitment to yourself.

If you're on vacation, or your routine is disrupted, choose another day or time within that week to stock up. Don't convince yourself you can get by. That rarely works.

Test: The store of your dreams is having a one-day, 70-percent-off-everything sale. The sale is the same day as your grocery store/stock-up day. What do you do?

Answer: Personally, I'd skip the sale. So should you. Sorry! I know that doesn't sound like much fun, but you have to decide what your priority is. There is nothing more important than providing yourself with healthy food choices.

Pick *your* grocery store/stock-up day and put it on your calendar.

The Importance of Food Prep

You also need a food preparation schedule. I spend about half an hour every Sunday and Monday cutting peppers, washing lettuce and fruit, shredding carrots, dicing tomatoes and preparing other vegetables. I also prepare and freeze healthy meals so they're on hand when I need them.

As I did while I was losing weight, I keep myself well supplied with these pre-made, healthy foods. Having them prepared and quickly available makes maintaining my hard-earned weight loss easy.

If I didn't prepare these foods in advance, I would never eat a variety of fruits, vegetables, and other healthy choices. Generally, they often take more time to prepare. When we're starving we're in no mood to chop, peel, and slice. That may be why, when I was at my peak weight, fruits and vegetables rarely appeared on my plate. No wonder I was undernourished and overweight!

I actually discovered the importance of food prep during my weight-loss journey. Some days I'd come home from school or work tired and frustrated. Making a salad was the *last* thing I'd want to do. When I was starving, taking the time to create something healthy and well balanced felt like forever. I wanted the easy and fast, rip-open-the-bag, stuff-it-in-my-mouth kind of food.

When I was starving and tired, it was too easy to just throw a huge serving of leftover pasta in the microwave. I'd eat much more pasta than I needed. If I had given myself the option of eating a large salad *with* the pasta, I would have been satisfied with fewer overall calories and had a more balanced and nutritious meal.

About 85 percent of the time, when I knew in advance that my roommates and I were going to order a pizza, I'd eat a big salad before it arrived. By the time the pizza was delivered, one large slice would almost always satisfy me. Low-fat, nutritious choices served to intercept my hunger!

However, there *were* times when I came home, saw a huge salad ready to eat, in the fridge and chose to go nuts on something like pizza. Remember, this *isn't* about being perfect.

At times, clients have healthy foods in the house, but don't want to take the time to prepare them. Much of what we are willing to do depends on our mood and our level of hunger. Frustration and stress make it very hard for us to be patient. Add hunger to that equation and we'll grab whatever we can get to eat, as fast as we can get it. So, even though the healthy foods are there, generally, we won't eat them unless we've made it easy.

Get the family involved. Make healthy food preparation a weekend project. Recruit one person to chop the veggies, another to wash fruit. Together decide what cookbook recipes to make for the week.

However you do it, whatever works for you, make sure those healthy, pre-made choices are available at all times.

I'm not suggesting my specific days—shopping on Sunday, chopping and freezing on Monday—will also work for you. You have to create your own schedule. But remember, it's very important for you to designate and stick to food prep days. It's critical to your weight loss that you *always* have healthy, easy-to-eat foods available when you need them.

Plan the Night Before

At bedtime, I evaluate my next-day schedule. Where do I have to be? How much free time will I have? Will I have any long meetings? Car trips? What time will I be home for dinner?

I develop a plan, choosing the foods I'll need to bring with me.

I used to run out of the house like a mad woman, a woman who remembered only her purse and her car keys.

Early in my weight loss, I hadn't yet discovered how important it was to design a food plan the night before.

Once, I had been at school for five hours without a bite to eat. (Remember I didn't always follow my own advice.) I had to be at work in thirty minutes. I was in my car on my way to work and I was starving. I hadn't brought any healthy snacks with me. When I arrived at work, rushing, I changed my clothes, and went in search of something to eat.

The hotel where I worked had a gift shop. I was desperate. I needed food fast. At the gift shop, I bought a handful of chocolate peppermint candies (starvation leads to bad choices) and ate all of them within a minute. Then I bought more. In total, I ate over twenty pieces of chocolate! (Hey, at ten cents a piece, dinner was a bargain.) I felt awful. Eating candy as a meal put me in a downward spiral and I continued to eat junk throughout the night.

That disastrous evening could easily have been prevented. After all, I'd already learned the importance of food preparation. I had healthy, low-fat choices waiting for me at home. But I hadn't brought any of them with me.

That experience made me realize that I had to develop a food-carrying strategy. One solution that worked for me was packing a whole wheat bagel with a small amount of peanut butter to carry with me on my most hectic day. I also learned to carry an emergency kit, which included fruit, a small baggie of healthy cereal, and a container of chopped veggies. I didn't necessarily eat them *all*, but knowing I had options provided a safety net.

Because I varied my choices I sometimes carried foods that needed to be kept cool. I bought an inexpensive cooler for storing yogurt, low-fat sandwiches (tuna, turkey), juice, cottage cheese, and low-fat cheese slices.

I *still* develop a next-day plan every night. I *still* carry foods with me and decide in advance what I'm having for dinner.

Make a list of healthy and appealing dinner choices and a list of breakfasts, lunches, and snacks. Give yourself *plenty* of options. Be prepared to fill up on fruits, vegetables, whole grains, and lean proteins.

When I first started developing a night-before plan, I'd pack a yogurt every day. After a few weeks, I couldn't tolerate the thought of *another* yogurt. Because I had limited my choice to yogurt, I burned out and started hitting the vending machines at school.

Variety is important. You should have at least five breakfast choices, fifteen dinner and lunch options, and twenty or more different snacks to choose from. If you find this too much of a challenge, purchase cookbooks focusing on healthy foods and create ideas based on several recipes. It's very important that you enjoy what you're eating.

My *successful* clients understand that you have to stay at least one step ahead of your hunger at all times. One client shared an interesting observation.

"Linda" pulled into a bank parking lot. Parked in the next space was a woman who was getting out of her car. Linda described her as "beautiful, fit, and healthy looking." This woman had a banana and a sandwich bag of crackers on her car seat.

"She inspired me," my client said. "I'll bet she's been eating healthy her entire life. She sure looked like someone who put time into herself!"

Seeing this fit woman traveling with healthy snacks confirmed the advice I had given Linda. By giving herself available, healthy food choices, this woman stayed ahead of her hunger and was fit and looked great. Linda saw for herself that you don't have to go hungry to reach your goal weight.

My healthy routines have evolved into habits. I no longer have to think about grocery-store day, food-prep day, or developing a food plan the night before. These are routines—part of my life.

Remember, examine your eating behaviors and create ways to make it easy to avoid the destructive ones.

Keep a Record

It was the last thing I wanted to do, but I made a decision to hold myself accountable for *anything* and *everything* I ate. In the past, I had played the "assuming" game. *I think I did pretty well today. I was in control. Now, how many pieces of cheese* did *I eat at the party? I don't think it was many*. Trying to evaluate my food behaviors from memory made it easy to forget the foods I didn't want to remember.

In the past I had gone on many commercial diet programs that had required me to record what I ate: I hated it! Three ounces of this, one medium-size piece of fruit, one-half slice of that. Writing it all down was time-consuming and tedious.

In the past it was all about tracking *food*. This time it would be about my tracking my food *behaviors*.

I would use the information I recorded to help me identify trouble spots. When did I eat most? Which foods did I have the most difficulty being around? Did I eat more on any particular day? *Was there a pattern to my behaviors?*

For eighteen months, I faithfully carried a little notebook. In it, I recorded my behaviors: good, bad, or terrible. In just a few months, a pattern started to emerge. I usually ate most after 4:00 P.M. If I started my day with something sweet I was "dangerous" around sugar for the entire day. If I ate a light lunch, I was in serious trouble from dinner through bedtime. And then there were Sundays. Sundays had an obvious pattern. That was my number one worst food-behavior day. I'd pick and eat to eat all day long. In addition to uncovering patterns, recording my food behaviors also helped to quickly identify my I-can't-stop foods.

It's important to note that I didn't record what I ate for the purpose of punishment or blame. *Oh, you ate too much pizza, Jennifer. I can't believe you did that, Jennifer! You know better than that!* I wasn't recording what I ate so that I could hear *that* voice. I did it in order to examine my behaviors, not to judge myself.

I learned a lot. I learned I don't dare keep I-can't-stop foods in my house. I learned that I need big, healthy lunches and a late-afternoon snack to be able to approach dinner in control. I learned I must eat before going to *any* social event where food is involved. I discovered I can't start my day with something sweet. For me, starting the day with sugar leads to disastrous food behaviors. By entertaining myself on Sunday, not allowing myself time for boredom eating, I can prevent Sunday "pig-out." I schedule walks with friends. I volunteer at a local animal shelter. I also filled some of my time by making Sunday food-prep day.

Because I focused on giving myself a reprieve from guilt, recording my behaviors around food became an enlightening, learning experience.

When I ask my clients to keep a food-behavior diary, some cringe. "Do I have to weigh and measure food? Can I have a big bagel for breakfast or should I eat one of those mini ones? How many ounces of meat should I have?"

They're used to the standard dieting approach. At first, clients seem confused when I say that I don't care about what or how much they eat. "Just focus on when and what types of foods you abuse," I tell them. "We're going to find out where, when, and why you eat the way you do."

Most clients seem relieved to learn that my weight-loss approach has nothing to do with being perfect. "Begin this weight loss by being yourself. In time we'll work on better food choices. For now, let's just focus on your normal food behaviors."

Today, I occasionally eat more than I need, or purchase one of my I-can't-stop foods. Now and then I engage in mindless eating. A return to these bad habits signals that I need to go back to recording my food behaviors. Doing this is always an eye-opener. It's amazing to see that eight years into my maintained weight loss, some of my old destructive food patterns are *still* with me. Examining and acknowledging them helps put me back on track.

Dedication

Most people know weight loss isn't rocket science and they suspect it's about more than just calorie reduction. But they may not know where to focus their weight-loss efforts.

I've explained how low-fat foods can actually sabotage your weight loss. I've encouraged you to eat five times a day. And I've provided you with strategies to help you survive social situations. We've discussed the importance of developing a routine: never missing a weekly trip to the grocery store, planning meals in advance, picking a "food-prep" day. I've suggested you record your food behaviors. We've covered enough information to make your head spin! It may seem like a lot to absorb, but believe me, this whole weight-loss process doesn't have to be difficult.

A lot of what it's about is getting focused. Your level of dedication to yourself will determine your likelihood of success. You must make your life-changing weight-loss goal your focus.

Habitualization

I threw that word in to see if you were paying attention.

There's a theory that if you eliminate a behavior, you have to replace it with another behavior or the behavior you eliminated will soon return. I'm asking you to replace bad food behaviors with good ones. If you do, the good food behaviors will become routine.

What routine behaviors do you engage in? Brushing your teeth? Doing laundry? Cleaning? If you have any routine behaviors, it's likely you don't think much about doing them. These behaviors, whatever they are, have become a natural part of your life. They're habits. Without much effort or resistance, you engage in these behaviors over and over again.

You can develop equally natural healthy food habits. Stay dedicated to healthy food behaviors and they *will* become habits.

I was successful at weight loss because I didn't give up. I was determined to set myself up for success. I didn't *try* to find time for the grocery store; I made a list of available days and times and *made* the time. Now, for me, stock-up day is a habit.

I methodically created daily food plans, until I realized I no longer had to think about doing it. Planning meals became automatic. Eating healthy foods and knowing how to make them became a habit. I recorded my eating patterns, when and why I ate, until eating in a sensible way became routine.

Because I developed a middle ground, I could give up being an all-or-nothing person.

My old thinking: *Well, I missed a trip to the grocery store. I might as well eat anything I can get. I stuffed myself with junk at the party. That does it. I quit! What's the point? I might as well just give up on myself.* This way of thinking did not work. I came to understand that "perfect" or "wrecked" were not my only weight-loss choices.

I no longer lectured myself with harsh words. I didn't punish myself or shame myself. Instead I learned to provide myself with words of encouragement. *Okay, Jennifer, eating that whole pie wasn't a great idea. What can I do next time that will prevent that overeating episode from happening again?*

Dedicate yourself to yourself. Make *yourself*, not food, your priority. Believe in yourself. And remember, permanent weight loss is about self-discovery.

5

Nobody's Business

Shhhhhh!

When you hear someone announce, "I'm trying a new diet," what's the first thing you think? Do you expect them to succeed?

You'll often hear cycle dieters use familiar words like "trying," "another," and "again." These words reflect the dieter's self-doubt and fear of failure. Though dieters who use these words want desperately to lose weight, their halfhearted language demonstrates that they don't really expect to succeed. Do you ever hear a superstar athlete using language like that?

"I'm going to *try* to win the game. I've got *another* pair of sneakers that just *might* help me win. If these sneakers don't help, I've heard there's *another* brand out there that's supposed to be pretty good." If you heard an athlete talking like this, would you expect him or her to win at anything?

Imagine a major athlete who believes that if he manages to win a race, it's only because of his sneakers. He doesn't believe in his own *ability* to win a race; it's the sneakers that pull it off. But, unfortunately the sneakers wear out quickly. They don't last very long. They may help him win once, perhaps even twice, but there are times when the sneakers don't even take him to the finish line. So he's in a constant search for the new, perfect pair of sneakers that will always make him a winner.

This scenario doesn't sound realistic because we all know major athletes win races because they believe in themselves and their ability. An athlete who has no confidence in himself and focuses instead on sneakers, expecting them to win the race for him, doesn't have a chance. Now substitute the word "diet" for "sneaker." If you fail on diets, it's because all of your energy is wasted, focusing on the diet. It should be focused on you.

Because I coach people one on one, it's impossible for clients to escape my attention. During our initial consultation, some people admit they are hesitant to work with me because they fear they will fail and disappoint me.

"I know my history," one client confided. "I try, but I'm impatient. If I don't lose fast enough, I quit." Clients often admit that with most commercial weight-loss programs, they can easily disappear under the radar, undetected. They can't do that in a one-on-one program and that intimidates them. They understand instinctively that my approach to weight loss puts the focus on them, not a diet.

Announcing we're on a diet really says, "I know I have a problem, and I just want you to know I'm addressing it."

There is a certain amount of vindication attached to our announcement. We're convinced everyone thinks we *should* be on a diet. When we make our declaration, we think we're doing what's expected of us. The announcement is intended to provide us with some guilt relief, even if it doesn't solve our problem.

What makes us think that we have to answer to anyone but ourselves?

In the past I was famous for my diet announcements. "I've heard about another, great new diet. I'm going to give it a *try!*"

My friends and family knew my history. I doubt they were ever surprised when, in time, I abandoned the diet and returned to my old eating habits. Short term I was willing to commit to a diet, no matter how awful it was. But I wasn't prepared to make a lifestyle change. At that point, I didn't even understand what a lifestyle change required. I was that insecure "athlete," still counting on those "sneakers" to win my race.

It took a while for me to see how my diet announcements sabotaged me. I eventually began to recognize the hazard they created.

At the beginning of my final, successful weight loss, I went out with my friends to a restaurant. When you're trying to lose weight, social situations are often difficult, and I felt very anxious.

After a night of partying, before heading home, my friends and I often would go somewhere for food. By the time we did, it was often late, very late. Sometimes I wasn't even hungry. At the time, I was in my twenties and still grossly overweight. But I was committed to changing my life. How could I do *that* unless I learned how to handle social situations? What behaviors sabotage me? Could I learn to coach myself through them?

In the past, I'd always announced—often at the table—that I was on a diet. Unfortunately, making that announcement set me up.

"Oh, come on Jen, one potato skin isn't going to kill you!"

They were absolutely right! *One* potato skin wouldn't kill me. What they didn't understand was, I wouldn't stop at one potato skin. By announcing I was on a diet, I invited my friends to encourage me to give in to the foods I wanted. I made what I ate or didn't eat the focus of attention.

I'm not blaming them. They had no idea what I was struggling with. How can the average person know what we go through? We either stick faithfully to our decision to lose weight, or we abandon it completely. It's the old black or white. So when someone with no food issues insists that "one won't hurt you," they have no way of knowing what one taste of a forbidden food can lead to: "That did it! I give up. I'm eating it all. I'll be perfect tomorrow."

When you play the weight-loss game it's easy to be talked into cheating. We want those forbidden foods *so* much, and deep down, we fear it's a matter of time before we blow it anyhow. We allow ourselves to be coaxed into having that first, diet-wrecking treat. Once we're no longer completely in control, we quickly become completely out of control. And as we're giving up, we're *already* making new, unrealistic promises to ourselves. "I'll get back on track tomorrow. One last night of all-I-can-eat fun, then I'll get serious again."

The announcement cycle, like the diet cycle, can seem never ending. But when my focus changed, I stopped making diet announcements. By focusing on yourself, *not* a diet, *you* can take *you* to the finish line—in private.

If you feel you have to offer an explanation for turning down weight-loss sabotaging foods, try this. Instead of saying, "I'm on a diet," say something like, "I've made a commitment to eating healthy. Thanks. I'm going to pass."

Stay positive. Keep yourself and your good-health goal your focus.

During my weight loss, I would happily have stampeded toward that plate of potato skins, trampling anyone in my path. But no one needed to know *that*. The part of me that longed for the potato skins didn't *care* about my body; the part of me that had taken control of my weight loss *did*.

If I sound like a person who was in conflict with herself, it's because I *was*. We chronic dieters live with an "angel" on one shoulder and a "devil" on the other. We either answer to our craving—*You want those potato skins. You love them. Everyone else is eating what they want, why should **you** suffer?* Or we answer to our guilt—*You were terrible last night! You must have gained five pounds! It's time to get back in control. Today is going to be perfect!*

This may sound weird, but I decided to stop listening to the devil *and* the angel voices and began to look for balanced, realistic answers within me. Operating in the extreme didn't work. Making diet announcements was another way of trying to *force* myself to be *perfect,* hoping that making a commitment to a diet out loud would help me to stay committed. It did just the opposite.

When I became confident, convinced I could get the fit body I wanted and keep that body, it was no longer important to announce my weight-loss goals to anyone.

Silence really *is* golden.

Tell Me Lies

One of my clients told me she was invited to her husband's boss's house for dinner. She didn't feel comfortable. How could she refuse their "famous" fried chicken without appearing rude? What could she do?

Desperate circumstances call for desperate measures. I told her to lie. Yes, lie.

I told her to focus on the healthy things that were being served. To comment on how wonderful the veggies or the salad looked, then to quietly share with the hostess the sad fact that she can't eat anything fried. "Your chicken looks delicious, but my cholesterol is through the roof. My doctor has given me *strict* instructions: no fried food."

No one will push any food when it threatens your health. It's an easy out. Who can argue with "doctor's orders"?

If telling a lie is out of the question for you, I can respect that. But, if that's the case, you may be too much of a goody-goody for me! Sinful habits call for sinful solutions!

Okay, okay, invent solutions that solve the problem, but leave your conscience clear. Just make sure your solution saves you from potential food-disaster situations.

For most of us, nothing during weight loss is more dangerous and difficult than being in foreign territory: a friend's house for dinner, a business luncheon, a family gathering, or any place where we fear temptation. If you're like me, then my advice is fib—fib away. Invent exotic diseases, religions with food restrictions, or fatty-meat aversion (developed since seeing the movie *Babe*). Whatever it takes, put your health first!

Food allergies are another great excuse. Some people use food allergies to explain weight gain. I recommend you make food allergy claims to *avoid* weight gain.

At a work appreciation party, managers bought pizza to reward us for good job performance. Eating healthy had already become my focus. Pizza had contributed to my downfall many times in my past. I knew from experience, one slice could easily lead to six. I knew I could control myself if the pizza had no cheese. Cheese had always been one of my I-can't-stop foods. During the party one of my co-workers saw me scraping the cheese from my slice of pizza.

"What are you doing?" she asked. "What's wrong with the cheese?" At that point, there were several, curious co-workers who seemed anxious to hear my answer.

No longer willing to announce to a lunchroom of fellow employees that I was trying to lose weight, I invented a creative answer.

"I'm allergic to certain types of cheese. Unless I know the ingredients, I can't eat it. I'll break out in huge hives." Oh, that was a good one! Pretty unappealing. Who wants to see their fellow co-worker turn into a giant hive?

"Wow, Jen, I didn't know that! That stinks!" Nobody tried to talk me out of avoiding the cheese.

From that day forward, I had to remember not to eat cheese in front of my co-workers. I deserved an Oscar for the "Dangerous Cheese" story!

Keep a sense of humor. Stay focused on your goal and remember that you're more likely to achieve healthy, successful weight loss if you make the process a personal and private experience.

6

You Gotta Get Moving!

But I Hate It!

Hate is a strong word. I was discouraged from using the word *hate* as a child, but when it came to exercise, I hated it. I hated the people that liked it. I hated hearing that it would help me lose weight. I hated the ads on television for the "beautiful body" health clubs that said I could look like the people in the ads. They intimidated me and I *hated* them, those people with the rock-hard stomachs, those people without an ounce of jiggle anywhere on their bodies.

The people in the exercise ads had to be crazy. Smiling while sweating? Makeup perfect, hair styled. Too phony for me! These were not people I'd associate with. I hated the whole idea. I wanted nothing to do with that scene. To hell with 'em!

My first exposure to exercise happened when I was about ten years old. By then I was four feet six and 150 pounds. My mother knew I was frustrated and was trying to help me lose weight. "Come on, Jennifer, we'll get some exercise." She took me to a women's health club. She had a sinister plan: she was going to make me move!

My mother weighed ninety pounds at the time. (Yes, you read correctly, ninety pounds.) Why did she want to go to this "place"? I had never seen her do any formal exercise, just earthy, crunchy back-to-nature stuff: cross-country skiing, gardening, planting trees, and walking in the mountains. So when she invited me along to this "fun" place, I didn't know what to expect. I had no idea that I was being set up.

I followed my mother into the building. I can only imagine how I looked—probably pretty cute. Chubby kids can be. I wore my hair in thick, long braids and Mom had bought me a perky, striped pink leotard with a white belt. Quite flattering, I'm sure—NOT!

I suspect some people were surprised we were mother and daughter. At ten, I weighed more than she did.

The place was crowded—women in tights everywhere! I remember feeling out of place because I was the only kid in the health club.

There were lots of machines! Big, scary looking machines that allowed you to walk, but stay in one place. Bicycles that you pedaled, but never traveled on. I wanted to leave. There were no other kids. This was not a fun place, not a place for me!

I was ready to tell my mom I wanted to leave but then . . . I saw it—the fun I'd been searching for—the machine of my dreams! Up on a platform was the one piece of equipment that intrigued me. I couldn't wait to give it a try!

I jumped on the platform, approached the machine and strapped myself in. A white belt encircled my waist. I leaned back and flipped a little silver switch, the machine shook me all over. This was great!

I remember yelling down to my mom, "Moooooooommmm, ttttthhhhhhhhiiissss iiiiiissssss fffffffunnnnn! IIII'mmmmmm sssssttaaayyyiiinnnnggg hheerrreee!"

Mom looked concerned. "Jen, why don't you try something else? I'm not comfortable with that particular machine. It's shaking you pretty hard. That can't be good for you! Besides, you should be using something that requires *you* to do the work, not the machine."

Work? That suggestion made me angry. She was trying to spoil my fun! Besides, why would this shaky machine be in the gym if it didn't help?

Looking back, she was right . . . again. Today you won't see that machine unless you visit an exercise equipment graveyard. God, how I wish that machine had been a fat burning breakthrough. Oh, for the good old days!

My mom and I went to the gym about three more times before I told her I didn't want to go anymore. I felt out of place and I didn't like exercise. She was very low pressure and never pushed me. I went back to playing with Barbie full-time.

It would be eleven years before I accepted the fact that exercise had to be part of a healthy lifestyle. By then, I knew I had no choice.

As a teenager, I wasn't completely sedentary. I played some sports: doubles tennis, one year of basketball. My friends were athletic, so I wanted to be as well. I didn't have to move as much for doubles tennis, I relied on my partner to make the fast moves. Basketball was more difficult. I *had* to run, therefore, I didn't play often. I was much too self-conscious to play most school sports. I felt out of place and awkward. Running was a tremendous effort. My athletic uniforms were tight and uncomfortable. My tennis skirt was special ordered. What seemed natural for the other girls was a struggle for me. As the years went on, I abandoned sports, and as a result, I got heavier.

By the time I was twenty-one years old, I was five feet two and over 200 pounds. Every weight-loss attempt had failed. I was sick of being dateless. I was tired of lying, creating excuses to get out of normal social activities, like going to the beach with my friends. I was sick of feeling my thighs rub together when I walked, and was sick of the way I had to dress to accommodate my weight. I was lonely and frustrated. I had hit rock bottom. As corny as this may sound, at rock bottom I finally decided that I liked myself too much to stay in such a state of misery.

I deserved better.

The Voice of Reason

When I began to examine my weight problem, from somewhere inside me, a very common-sense, rational voice I hadn't heard before said, "Jennifer, you have the power to change your life. You can continue to be miserable or you can lose weight."

I'd talked to myself before, but I'd never spoken to myself without using judgmental language. This voice wasn't telling me what I'd done wrong, it was telling me I could change my life and for the first time I believed that this was a possibility.

A New Beginning

I began my brand-new life on a bitterly cold day by lacing up my old sneakers and going for a walk. It was that simple, but it wasn't easy.

I was in horrible shape, breathless when I walked up stairs. After playing "chase" with neighborhood children one day, I nearly collapsed. Every time I got the chance, I sat down. I was always tired.

So why did I start with a walk? It was something I *could* do. In the past I'd never exercised during *any* attempts to lose weight. Every expert said exercise helped with weight loss. I was determined to find out if that was true. Would moving more help me lose weight or feel better about myself? I had to try.

I huffed and puffed for the entire five minutes. I was reminded why I never wanted to exercise! I *hated* it. Hated it. Catch 22. I hated exercise because it made me uncomfortable in countless ways. My inner thighs chafed when I walked. Only baby powder soothed the pain. My knees hurt. My muscles ached and so did my back. I was self-conscious about how I looked. The list went on and on. But I knew everything that bothered me could be changed if I lost weight and got in shape.

I had the power.

I cursed the cold every step of the way. My face burned from the wind. Even my dog wanted no part of it. She kept looking up at me as if to say, "Are you crazy? I liked you better curled up on the couch watching talk shows."

In the past, I would have taken my dog's advice. But this time I wasn't going to create excuses. I was determined to take that "first step."

But it's never *that* easy, is it?

Make Me Invisible

I thought, "What must I look like to all the people looking out their windows in this condominium complex? Are they laughing? Do they think I look huge? Are my horrible workout clothes giving them a chuckle?"

I was far from stylish in my extra-large, hot pink windbreaker, oversized sweatpants, and high-top sneakers. I desperately wanted to turn back, back to the security of my home. No one judged me there. It was safe. It was the familiar place where I was comfortable being uncomfortable.

Like most overweight people who begin to exercise, I was very self-conscious. We feel like all eyes are on us. I imagined people watching me wondering, "What does she think *she's* doing?" Or, worse yet, "Why bother?"

Self-consciousness comes from being insecure. Because of my body, I *was* painfully insecure. I wanted a new body, but what if, while trying to get a new body, I would make myself the target of jokes? That thought terrified me. In the past I had been called "Fatso" and other names that were meant to wound, and they did. Pain can immobilize us, if we let it.

Cruel people can inflict pain. But you aren't the only person they'll target. People get teased for a lot of different reasons. And, deep down, the people who torment others have their own list of problems. Surrendering your happiness to people who enjoy wounding you is like putting a bully in charge of your life. Some people are mean, but they are not in the majority.

Unfortunately, those of us who are unhappy with our weight are so insecure we think the whole world is evaluating us, judging us. The truth is we're hypersensitive to the negative feedback because we're often making those harsh judgments about ourselves. What we imagine people are thinking about us is actually a reflection of what *we're* thinking. It goes back to our need to be perfect. If we're not perfect, we tell ourselves we're worthless and we've failed.

I was constantly evaluating other people's bodies, making unfavorable comparisons of my body to theirs. I assumed (in fact I was sure) people were doing the same thing to me. That made it extremely difficult to get beyond my self-conscious fear and embarrassment.

Gradually, I changed my thinking. I knew I had to. This negative thinking was undermining my efforts.

Was it possible, I began to ask myself, that people looking out their windows weren't putting me down? I imagined them saying, *Good for her. She's doing something about her weight.* Maybe they were thinking they should be out walking, too. Or maybe—and this is very hard for many overweight people who are painfully self-conscious about their weight to believe—they were paying *no* attention to me at all!

With each positive step my attitude continued to change. For the first time the "balance of power" had shifted. In the past all the power rested in whatever diet I was on. *Would the **diet** succeed? Would the* *diet provide the "secret" of success?* This time the power was coming from **me.** Nothing could stop me. It was a new beginning and not even my insecurities were going to discourage me. I was on a roll.

What a Feeling!

My initial five-minute walk gradually expanded to ten minutes, four times a week. Soon, I was walking for twenty minutes, five times a week.

I began to notice small changes in my body. The changes inspired me to work harder, and working harder got easier as I continued to get in better shape. By April I was down two sizes. I had lost my first twenty pounds! I felt empowered. I felt strong for the first time in my life.

There were no hills in the neighborhood where I walked. Having hit a plateau with my weight, I was (my body was) getting used to the walk and needed more of a challenge. For two months, my clothes— which were the best gauge for my progress—fit the same. They weren't getting looser. I needed to see more results in order to feel motivated.

Instead of becoming discouraged, I accepted the truth. To continue losing weight, I had to work harder. I bought a used treadmill and tried the "hill" program. This program was more challenging than the flat walk. Soon, I started making progress again. My body started changing. By not giving up, by trying harder, I broke the plateau! I continued to look better and feel stronger.

My self-esteem continued to grow. I was ready to join the local YMCA. In its catalogs, the people pictured didn't look like perfectly fit, beautiful people. They looked normal. The "Y" wasn't selling beauty. I liked that.

Walking into that Y for the first time was one of the hardest things I've ever done. I felt I didn't belong and suspected everyone there believed that about me as well. I imagined everyone thinking, "What is *she* doing here?"

My insecurities were building up again. The negative voices came back. They had always succeeded in overpowering me when I was most vulnerable. This time, I wouldn't let them win. I had never wanted weight loss this badly before. In the past I would debate with myself:

Should I continue exercising?

Oh, why bother? I'll look ridiculous and it won't do any good.

But I hate the way I look. I hate my life. I've got to start some-where. I can't stay this way forever.

But nothing you do is going to help. Even if you start, it'll take forever. Why bother?

This time I didn't play that game with myself. I didn't debate the pros and cons with the negative, hopeless part of me. This time I wasn't willing to take "you can't succeed" for an answer.

For the very first time, I was determined that there would be no more self-defeating debates. The fitness choice was the *only* choice, and it was for life. At last I allowed myself to believe the fitness choice was a realistic and attainable goal.

Just because I had this new level of determination, doesn't mean it was easy.

The gym environment was so new. There were lots of people: fit people, older people, overweight people, kids, moms, and dads. I was nervous.

I met with the fitness trainer who suggested I warm up on the exercise bike. She set the program on level one (the lowest level) for twelve minutes. After three minutes I nearly keeled over. How discouraging! I could walk for forty minutes, biking for twelve should be a breeze! At the time, I didn't realize that an entirely different group of muscles that hadn't been used before were screaming, "Why? Why!"

I had to stop pedaling. I felt like a failure. All my hard work meant nothing. I couldn't even ride the bike for three minutes. The trainer couldn't believe I had to stop, which made me feel even worse. Some-how I had overestimated my progress. What followed was the return of the negative voices. *Who am I kidding? You're an embarrassment.* At that point, the easiest thing for me to do, the thing I *wanted* to do, was to walk out. Quit.

No!

That was the old Jennifer, quick to throw in the towel.

Leaving the gym, I sat in my car, thinking long and hard. *Should I quit?*

No.

The next day—no matter what—I was going to go back and ride the bike for *five* minutes. That was how I had begun with walking. I would do the same with the stationary bike.

My new plan was to approach every activity that way; start as slowly as possible and work my way up.

Within three months I had reached a new level of fitness. I was now walking for forty minutes and, on other days, biking for thirty. My determination was paying off. The trainer and I had become friends. I was a gym "regular."

In a few more months, more pounds and inches disappeared. I gathered enough courage to try a step aerobics class.

At first, it was awful. I was, by far, the most uncoordinated person in the class! When Larry, the instructor, stepped up I stepped down. When the class faced right, I faced left. I wanted to run out of the class with my towel draped over my head!

Larry sensed my humiliation and asked if I would allow him to show me some of the moves after class.

Under his guidance, I practiced and got better. I now not only walked and biked, I also did a mean step aerobics class!

For only *one year* I had been focused and determined and was already well on my way to becoming the person I knew I could be.

Can It Be?

Then the strangest thing happened. Not *one*, but *two* instructors told me I had great form. "You should consider teaching." *Should consider teaching?* Ha! Were they kidding? This can't be real! Me, the girl who was afraid to walk in public, become an aerobics instructor?

At that point I was sixty pounds closer to my seventy-pound weight-loss goal. I felt like a new person. I was proud of myself because I hadn't allowed any obstacle to stand in my way. I was able to keep up with any aerobics instructor. I was capable of maintaining rhythm. I knew the moves.

Okay, maybe I could teach.

I set out to become certified as an aerobics instructor. I was determined to be a darn good aerobics instructor: one who could change people's lives, the way Larry had changed mine.

The aerobics instructors who encouraged me provided me with a list of workshops I would be required to take to become certified. Without hesitation, I enrolled in the classes, and three months later, got my certification.

Don't panic. I'm not suggesting you become an aerobics instructor. I became one because, at this point, I was beginning to think a career in health and fitness could be a choice for me. And as it turned out, it was. Encouraging others became my goal.

As an instructor, I quickly saw that the people participating in the classes were of various fitness levels. There were overweight people, older people, beginners, and athletes. Seeing such a mix of body types wasn't what I expected. Before viewing a class as an instructor, it had seemed to me that classes were nearly always filled with extra-fit, tight bodies. I'd always imagined myself being the oddball, trapped on the set of *Flashdance*. I learned how untrue that actually was. Typically, an aerobics class is filled with an assortment of body types. But, even if you accept that fact, the key lies in feeling comfortable. If you are prepared to begin, but feel a little intimidated, find a health club that offers classes for beginners. Also, keep in mind, everyone is uncoordinated at first. If you feel self-conscious, position yourself in the very back of the class while you're working on becoming familiar with the basic steps. I guarantee, if you stick with it, your skills will improve with every class.

Eventually, I decided to move on to another coaching level. The idea of inspiring people one on one appealed to me. I knew from experience that there was a need for sensitive people in the fitness industry. Most people enter the field already fit. They've never had a weight problem. *But I had been there.* Personal experience had taught me that, when setting a stationary bike for a beginner—particularly an overweight beginner—three minutes, not twelve, was a realistic goal. I also knew how intimidating starting a fitness program could be. For us, the focus has to include building confidence, not just muscles.

Exercise is crucial if you really want to give yourself the life-improving gift of fitness. Investing in exercise has many benefits. It will motivate you to make better food choices. It also helps you evaluate potentially destructive food behavior in a different way.

"I walked for an hour today and worked up quite a sweat! Do I *really* want to cancel out the calories burned from my walk on *two* cookies?"

Okay, there *were* those occasional times when I said, "Heck, yes! Sounds like a fair trade-off to me!" (Remember, I wasn't perfect.) But exercise boosted my self-esteem. It was the key to staying focused.

Set a Goal

When I have clients who fail to exercise regularly, they find it difficult to lose weight. Their lack of commitment to exercise reflects a lack of commitment to themselves.

Visualize a baseball diamond. Imagine your weight-loss journey as a trip around that diamond, with each base representing a specific fitness goal. Failing to include exercise makes the trip feel like this:

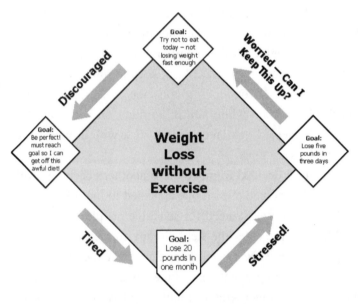

How long before the next diet?

You drag slowly toward first base (maybe that first base goal is to lose five pounds in three days). Getting there is a struggle. You have little energy. It's a rough trip. Consequently, once there, you lack the motivation to head toward your next unrealistic goal, which waits for you at second base. But somehow you manage to get there. Then you begin to crawl toward third. You're discouraged. Your energy level is zero. You're primed to give up. *I'll eat whatever—who cares? Home plate looks miles away. I'll never make it.*

If you are consistently including exercise in your weight-loss plan, your trip around the baseball diamond feels like this:

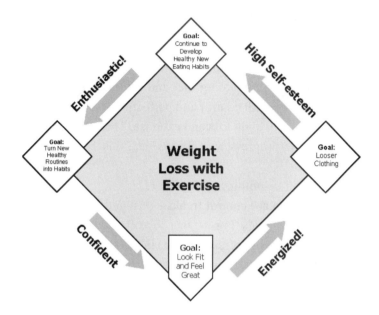

You're energized as you approach first base. Rounding second base you notice an increase in self-esteem. As you're sprinting toward third, treating yourself better feels more and more natural. Sliding into home plate and scoring that run is easy.

If you make exercise part of your "trip" around the weight-loss diamond, everything else will fall into place. You'll love the feeling of confidence it gives you. Try it. Start slowly. Begin by setting very small goals.

Once my clients have exercised for more than six months on a regular basis, exercise almost always becomes part of their lives.

Does walking for five minutes a day sound overwhelming? Make it three minutes. If you can handle more, do more. The point is, don't go to extremes. I started with five minutes. Today, I run and lift weights. I exercise five times a week. Not because I have to, but because I love it. My energy level is off the charts. *Me*—the girl who used to sit on the sofa all day! My self-esteem has never been higher. My body is healthy and trim. It's the body the very overweight me so desperately wanted. And exercise helped give it to me. Granted, it took time. But if I hadn't persevered, that time would have gone by anyhow and I'd still be on the sofa eating junk food, waiting for my life to change.

You don't have to be perfect. I exercised less during some weeks than others, but I never quit. I set my own *realistic* timetable. I never beat myself up when, on some days, I chose not to exercise.

I abandoned my *all-or-nothing* mentality. I had been all or nothing in everything I did regarding diet and exercise. That's common. Many clients wrestle with control and perfection issues. You must not bring those issues to weight loss and exercise. They'll only set you up for failure. A little progress will always take you farther than a big defeat.

Are you an all-or-nothing personality?

Those of us who are control freaks—past and present—regularly strive for unrealistic goals. For us, one slip often triggers total defeat. Some of my clients were exercise junkies in their pasts. But they never approached exercise in a healthy way because they never allowed themselves to slip. It was always all or nothing.

We chronic dieters handle exercise and food in similar ways. We're compulsive. If we eat *that* cookie or skip *that* walk it's all over. We've failed. And we go into that old familiar cycle: self-disgust, anger, sadness, and defeat. We leap from *perfect* to *out of control,* with nothing in between.

If you're an all-or-nothing person, a perfectionist, this will sound familiar. You've probably set unrealistic goals. You're probably very hard on yourself. Everything is either black or white. Control is everything. The smallest setback equals failure.

I succeeded when I let go of my rigid, all-or-nothing way of thinking. No more of the quick-fix mentality. But sticking to an exercise routine was still hard to do. Some days I didn't want to exercise. Some days I wondered why I was still exercising at all. I wasn't seeing results fast enough so why bother?

But, to my surprise, I loved the way exercise made me feel. I became aware that I was no longer exercising for vanity, I was exercising for sanity. Exercise had proven to be a major stress reliever. For me, exercise rechannels nervous energy. By exercising, I learned to recycle stress-producing energy. I used that negative energy to propel me toward my positive fitness goal. Exercise also replaced a destructive behavior. Instead of using food to relieve stress, I was now relieving it with exercise.

Let's face it, after comforting ourselves with food, guilt usually kicks in and we actually end up with increased stress. After exercising, even a little bit, I feel I've done something positive. And feeling positive makes it a lot easier to stay on track.

For us, the solution lies in accepting that there's a middle ground, a large, comfortable gray area that lies between black and white. If the only choice you've given yourself is not exercising at all, consider that exercising even *one time* in a week represents a positive step toward success.

What Works for You?

Often, clients hope to apply my exercise regime to their own life. "What do you do, Jennifer?" When I tell them I occasionally teach aerobics, run four to five miles a day or lift weights, they look discouraged. They usually say something like, "I could never do that!" or "I'd collapse if I tried that!"

Keep in mind, it took me *years* to get to this fitness level. If I had begun my exercise attempts by running, I, too, would have collapsed.

One of my friends is a marathon runner. She is a role model for fitness and health. If I had asked her what she did for exercise in the beginning of my personal quest to lose weight and she had said she ran ten miles a day, my self-sabotaging voice would have said, "Jennifer, you could never even come close to running for *one* minute. Why bother?" But what she did wasn't important. What mattered was what *I* could realistically do. I had to set *my own* exercise goals.

When it comes to fitness, age is *not* a factor but it can be used as an excuse. I often hear, "Jennifer, you were twenty-one when you started exercising. I'm in my thirties (forties, fifties, sixties, seventies). I can't do what you did."

I've heard it countless times. My usual response is, "What you're telling me is you can't take a five-minute walk? Because that's how I started. My body was just as out of shape as yours."

Do me a favor. Go to a health club and observe an aerobics class for seniors. I was blown away by some of these people—better bodies than I'll ever have! They're inspirational!

I've met some people in their fifties who seem more like eighty-year-olds. I've met people in their seventies who seem more like forty. Besides helping with weight loss, studies show exercise helps people stay youthful.

People often quit before they give exercise a fair chance. If you don't believe me, visit a health club in January, February, or March. The place will be filled with people. Then visit again in April, May, or June. The place will be a lot less crowded. Granted, the urge to exercise outdoors is the reason for some of the decrease, but for others, it was because they had failed to see quick results.

Don't get discouraged if you don't enjoy exercise right away. For the first few months I hated exercise, too. On a daily basis I asked myself if it was really worth it. I stuck it out because I repeatedly told myself it could only get easier. It did. As I became more fit, exercise became more enjoyable.

Don't let a few weeks or a couple of months determine if you're going to love or hate exercise. Be consistent with a basic walking program or whatever you feel you will commit yourself to.

I assure you, if *I* can learn to love it, anyone can!

Check with your doctor first, but walking is the way I got started. It is low impact and almost any beginner can walk for five minutes.

Remember, starting out with a bang can lead to a flat tire. Start with a goal that's realistic and work from there.

My clients are often confused when we set goals. "Jennifer, I used to walk all the time! I'll start this week by walking all seven days for an hour!" What I say next often surprises them. "How about keeping it down to four times this week for thirty minutes?"

Remember, start with what's realistic. We're all-or-nothing people. If my client had not met her seven-day, one-hour walking goal, she would have felt as if she failed. It would have been harder for her to start again the following week.

Set goals you can reach and you will succeed!

Winning with a B+

Did I mention the *very* best benefit of exercise? You'll experience it during *and* after weight loss. No, it isn't just the increased esteem, or increased energy. It's not the fact that you'll develop more confidence, or that you'll become more fit. It's even better.

I was thrilled to discover that I could get away with eating more food than I had *ever* eaten during any weight-loss attempt. Exercise dramatically increased my metabolism. My body was (on average) efficiently using 1,600 to 1,800 calories, an amount that kept me satisfied. I never felt deprived. I wasn't suffering, *and* I was losing weight!

My diet history? Lose weight by restricting food intake. It had included little or no exercise. This meant that in *my* personal fireplace there were no flames. (Remember the "Light My Fire" chapter?) It consisted of a few, weak, barely-burning coals. Even with reduced food consumption, my weight-loss progress was slow. Discouraged, I always abandoned the diet and returned to my old destructive ways.

Then I became *determined* to change the way my fireplace burned fuel. I wanted a bonfire, and I knew that in order to build one, I had to stay *consistent* with an exercise program. I had to stay committed. I couldn't be dedicated to exercise for one week, then skip it completely the next—not if I was serious about building a more efficient metabolism.

I had become aware that weight loss represented a mental as well as a physical challenge. I accepted the truth: it wasn't realistic to expect "perfect." I was human; I would make mistakes.

Occasionally I would eat too much pizza, too many french fries, or half a bag of my favorite neon-yellow cheese puffs. I might eat more than I need, while out with a friend, or inhale a large candy bar.

Successful weight loss doesn't demand an A+ eating score. In fact, A+ is the score that most often results in failure. You are much more likely to win with a B+.

Clients are often shocked when they learn how much they can eat and still lose weight. But they can *only* do that if they stick to an exercise program.

One client (I'll call her "Maggie") continues to enjoy three slices of pizza weekly with her family on "pizza night." In the past she had always felt obliged to give up pizza. None of her diets encouraged eating three slices of pizza a week. Excluded from pizza night, she'd watch as her family ate one of her favorite foods, while she consumed an uninteresting frozen diet meal. Needless to say, she was always very anxious for her diets to end.

Over time, she couldn't handle being excluded from the pizzafest. Maggie eventually rebelled, abandoned the diet, and ate *five* slices of pizza at one sitting to make up for lost time. Sound familiar? We never lose *all* our destructive food behaviors. At least I haven't. But a life-long commitment to some kind of regular exercise gives you room when you have an, "Uh-oh, I really wish I hadn't eaten that" day. If you derail *after* you have increased your metabolism through exercise, the occasional damage you do won't succeed in undermining your weight loss.

7

Where's Your Head?

Is Success in Your Future?

Successful weight loss is about breaking old, bad habits and replacing them with new, healthy ones. It also requires a commitment and complete honesty. Healthy weight loss also requires *patience*. Because we chronic dieters have been conditioned to believe that fast weight loss represents success, we react with panic to the suggestion that we lose weight slowly. We know we can make that short sprint to the diet finish line, but that long weight-loss marathon . . . ? We don't believe we can win that one. When we finally decide to make weight loss our focus, we want the results to be *immediate*. "Why is this taking so long?" my clients sometimes ask. "I need to lose this disgusting fat *now*!"

If you aren't prepared to allow yourself as much time as you need to reach your weight-loss goal in a healthy way, then you aren't ready for my approach. Nothing of quality can be produced fast, including a fit body.

I observe common behaviors in people who are not ready to lose weight, and I hear a familiar language.

Most people sign up for my program with the best of intentions. But some arrive late for our first session, or not at all. They cancel appointments because of other commitments, or regularly forget our scheduled meeting day. They really *do* want to lose weight, but other things regularly distract them. They easily lose their focus.

They convince themselves that they've accomplished something simply because they've made a commitment to a weight-loss program, even if they don't actually follow through.

I understand. I used to buy workout tapes and would watch them while I sat on the couch, eating popcorn. "When I'm in better shape," I would tell myself, "I'm going to try some of those moves." The tapes became dust collectors.

How do you *feel* about weight loss? Do you feel compelled to explain why you can't lose weight? If you do, what purpose do those "explanations" serve? Do they provide relief? Vindication? Do they free you of responsibility or guilt?

The fact is that you don't owe *any* explanations for your weight to *anyone* but yourself. If you can live with, "I'm not ready to do what it takes to lose weight," then accept that, and focus on the things that are more important to you. I'm serious. I didn't lose weight until I was ready. I chose to do it when I made weight loss my most important goal. Once I made that decision, nothing, *nothing* could stand in my way. Losing weight was my choice. It is not a choice you can make until you are ready.

You have the right to stay overweight forever, if that's where you want to be. I'll bet no one ever told you *that* before. You're free to give up your weight-loss struggle. You really only have two choices; achieve the body you've always wanted or stay overweight. Engaging in a defeating, lifelong struggle with your weight should not be included in your choices.

But, if you *do* prefer to keep a lifelong struggle at the top of your list of choices, read the following personal experiences for the sure-fire ways to do it.

Self-diagnosis

Do you believe certain foods cause you to gain weight? Are you convinced that because you crave certain foods, you're addicted to them?

Consciously or unconsciously, do you feel obliged to offer an explanation for your weight problem? If there was no guilt attached to being overweight in our society, if "fat" was beautiful, would you *still* feel it was important to announce that you had a food allergy or addiction? Did you ever know a fit person who felt they had to justify their eating of a candy bar or a donut?

It's very tempting to provide explanations for our cravings. Personally, I love sweet treats, bread, pasta, and crackers. I *love* most carbohydrates. I never actually believed I was addicted or allergic to them. I knew I simply loved the taste and had a tough time stopping when I ate too much. And when I did eat too much, I gained weight. In an attempt to explain my eating, I offered other self-diagnosed reasons for my weight problem. "I must have a deficiency in something cookies provide. I crave them."

Since coaching others, I see why people rely on self-diagnosis. Declaring that an "addiction" or "deficiency" or any other self-diagnosed reason is responsible for weight helps people explain their inability to control their craving for certain foods.

I crave my favorite foods because they're my *favorite foods*. These foods provide fast, tasty gratification. Fortunately, I've finally learned how not to overeat them.

My self-diagnosing clients are most often convinced that they have either a food allergy or a food addiction. If you have scientific proof that you have an allergy or addiction to a specific food, then your goal has to be to stay away from that food.

It's curious that our self-diagnosed allergies always cause a weight-gain reaction. Most allergic reactions result in things like hives, short-term respiratory problems, or rashes. An allergic reaction often produces a considerable level of discomfort and the victim goes to great lengths to avoid that food in the future. But we often find ourselves eating these allergy-producing foods again and again. Oops!

If you eat a healthy, balanced diet and are physically active *on a regular basis* but gain weight for unexplained reasons, then perhaps you *do* have a medical problem that needs attention. This should be professionally evaluated. But this is where it's critical to be absolutely honest with yourself.

At my peak weight, I was an Emmy-winning self-diagnoser. If I ate a bag of potato chips it was because my salt levels were low. If I ate a large amount of chocolate it was because my hormone levels were out of whack. Had I ever been given this information by a medical professional? Heck no. But it sure did sound good coming from me! My delivery was perfect.

Also, I loved using the word "metabolism." Like a scientist, I threw the *metabolism* word around. My failed weight-loss attempts were always because of my "slow metabolism." How unfair! Everyone else in my family was blessed with a *speedy* metabolism. Not poor Jennifer! No matter how hard I tried, my "snail-like" metabolism hindered my weight-loss attempts. I had convinced myself that *it* alone explained why I was forty pounds overweight by age fourteen.

In my ultimate-fantasy scenario, a prestigious doctor would administer a test, an obscure metabolic test, that when the results arrived would cause the doctors and nurses to gather around me. I would be declared a "medical mystery." I would be labeled "the girl with no metabolism": the unfortunate girl who—though she eats only one tiny sandwich at a time—packs on the pounds; the girl that—though she goes on long, long, arduous walks—never loses weight.

Then *everyone* would understand. Finally I would be declared innocent of the worst crime in the entire universe: eating too much. I would be free to live my life without guilt.

At that point in my life, I wasn't ready to take responsibility for my eating and exercise habits. And I certainly didn't know how to do it without blame.

It would still console me to hear some doctor say, "I understand weight loss is tougher for *you*, Jennifer. You have a unique metabolism." It would be comforting to imagine someone saying they know my struggle with weight has been difficult. Although those words might provide some consolation, they wouldn't provide an excuse for weight gain today.

There *are* people with diagnosed medical reasons for weight gain. I've worked with a few. Their medical condition makes weight loss particularly difficult. They're under the care of a doctor and working to get well. They're doing everything in their power to succeed. They don't want this medical "reason" to become an excuse. In spite of their additional problem, they're determined to achieve their goal!

When I gave up looking for excuses for my weight problem, I was left with questions about my eating habits that I could not explain. That was when I considered that maybe my body didn't measure the intake of food the way most other people's bodies did. That was when I considered that perhaps my hunger meter was broken.

So what distinguishes my broken hunger meter observation from a self-diagnosis?

I *am* convinced that *our* mechanism for measuring how much food we need is faulty. Our hunger meter is broken. I had to explain my overeating to myself, and that's how I did it. Did a *doctor* ever tell me I had a broken hunger meter? No. You will probably *never* hear a doctor use the words "hunger meter." So you *could* call my explanation for overeating a self-diagnosis. But this is the difference: I *knew* I had a problem in the way I related to food. I *knew* that I didn't eat like people who had no food issues. While I *knew* weight loss would change my life and I *knew* creating excuses for my weight was only going to keep me overweight and miserable, I could not find an explanation for my eating patterns. Nothing made sense until I considered the fact that my body and brain did not *measure* my food intake the way other people's brains and bodies did. When I *considered* the fact that this might be true, I now had a problem I could focus on and address.

Let's go back to the car analogy. Let's pretend the gas gauge on my car is broken. My car is either out of gas, leaving me frantic and stranded, or it has fuel overflowing from the gas tank, which floods the engine and creates a potential safety hazard. There's no in between. Because my car doesn't work right, I'm always making excuses for it: "Oh, gosh, when I use *that* gasoline, my car never works right," or "I didn't pump *that* much gas into the tank! Why is it overflowing?"

Instead of working hard to provide acceptable *excuses* for my car's broken fuel gauge, I should try to determine *what's* causing my car to perform this way. What do the people with efficiently running cars have that I *don't* have? Wait a minute! They rely on their car's fuel gauge! It tells them when their tank is full, empty, and anywhere in between. What a concept! I want one of those! Uh-oh—mine doesn't work. Can I learn to function with a faulty one? *Yes!*

I learned how to lose weight, and to keep it off in spite of the fact that I still have a "faulty fuel gauge."

That's the difference between an excuse and a reason. A *reason* for behavior provides insights that help us *change* the behavior. An *excuse* gives us the opportunity to keep on doing exactly what we're doing.

Overeat, Who Me?

"It's not fair!" I would often exclaim. "I eat one sandwich, I gain five pounds! My brother eats whatever he pleases, and look at him! He's a walking skeleton!"

No one—but me—knew the truth. When I ate at a friend's house, I would stuff my face. While baby-sitting, I'd privately polish off a block of cheese and a box of crackers. I'd barter for food with the kids at school or stop at the convenient mart on the way home. I had my own private food relationship and no one needed to know.

My mother and brother ate in a controlled way. They stopped after one sandwich while I continued to eat long after I was stuffed. My brother rode his bike. My mother walked. I rarely joined them; I was a "sitter." Occasionally I rode my bike but I liked sitting better than being active.

It took several years before I was ready to be honest with myself. I was more comfortable being angry about my weight and complaining about my "bad luck": the only overweight member of a thin family. I was not prepared to confront the fact that I ate too much and moved too little. That prospect felt embarrassing, painful, and overwhelming. Getting honest with myself was one of the hardest things I have ever done.

It's tough, even painful, but taking ownership of your behavior is the make-or-break issue in weight loss. It is very important. When you take ownership of your food behaviors, that's when your life will begin to change.

A red flag goes up when I hear, "Jennifer, I'm doing *everything* right! Why can't I lose weight?"

These people aren't being completely honest with me or themselves. We don't deny our food behaviors on purpose. Part of us believes that we don't eat enough to gain weight. The problem is we do much of our eating in a mindless state. It isn't until I ask clients to record what they eat that they become conscious of their excessive food intake. But, in extreme cases, even that doesn't help. When all else fails, I sometimes suggest a person in eating denial seek professional medical advice. If, as they claim, they're exercising four to five times a week and eating a balanced, calorie-reduced diet, then I'm stumped. Perhaps a doctor can explain why they're not losing weight.

Most often they're simply not ready to face the fact that they're in denial. Again, there is nothing wrong with this; it's simply not their time to focus on weight loss.

"I'm Damaged"

Some people believe weight loss is harder for them due to circumstances that existed early in their life. I've been told that certain childhood events cause irreversible damage resulting in chronic bad food behaviors. For example, some people are convinced that their lack of control comes from years of being told to "clean" their plate.

"Wendy" was convinced weight loss could not happen for her. "Jennifer, I still eat large portions and I clean my plate because I was forced to as a child. I don't think I'll ever get over that programming."

"Ben" told me he was overweight because he grew up in a large family where people competed for food. At mealtime, everyone fought for their share. When the breadbasket hit the table it was chaos, hands everywhere. He learned at a very young age to hoard food, hide it in closets and dressers. He believes that's why he rushes through meals and overeats in private.

If someone has had a traumatic experience, and they believe that is responsible for their weight problem, then the event should be dealt with by a therapist. *The more pressing issue must be dealt with before attempting weight loss because weight loss will never be their primary focus.* If there seems to be an underlying, bigger problem, weight loss will not solve it.

There is a major difference between being told to "clean your plate" and a *life-altering* trauma that results in a person habitually seeking comfort in food. Ask yourself, *is my reasoning valid? Does an event really explain why I can't lose weight?*

If the answer to these questions is yes, then consider that the event currently has control of how you deal with your weight. Does it deserve that power? Your priority should be finding an answer to that question and a resolution for that problem.

Searchers

Some people come to me in search of reasons why they're overweight. They *think* they know why they're overweight, but they're not *sure*. "Jennifer, I *think* I'm overweight because I was teased in first grade.

That's when I believe my self-esteem was destroyed. Or *maybe* it was because I was told to clean my plate as a kid because other kids were starving in foreign countries. Or *maybe* it's because . . . "

The "why" is their focus. If they can only determine the "why," they *believe* their weight problem will be solved.

I'm a former searcher. At my peak weight (over 200 pounds) I'd confide to close friends that I thought my parents' divorce caused my weight gain. Looking back, it may have been somewhat responsible because I was stressed and depressed. But I was very overweight *before* the divorce and very overweight long *after* the divorce. Eventually, when I provided the divorce excuse, I began to listen to myself. It no longer sounded believable, even to me. I realized I couldn't keep blaming this event.

I was beginning to change. As I changed, my focus changed. Providing reasons for my weight became less important. Losing weight became the most important thing to me. How were excuses going to get me where I wanted to go?

Life throws the occasional curve ball; it happens to everyone. People with no weight problems have had traumatic events in their lives, too. The issue is not whether tough things have happened to you; the question is how do you deal with those events? How much power over your life do you choose to give them?

Every new day provides a clean slate. Imagine yourself dutifully recording your "reasons for failure" on your slate every morning. "This happened to me. That happened to me." That's what you *have* to do to *keep* yourself in an "I can't do it because. . . ." mode. "I can never lose weight or have a fit body because. . . ."

Now imagine writing "I *can* do it. I *can* lose weight!" on that clean slate first thing every morning. Declare yourself a "winner." Make winning possible. If you can declare yourself a winner, you *can* tackle your weight.

Do you think of yourself as wrecked, damaged, or abnormal? Then do *whatever* it takes to find out why you feel that way. But, if you can say, "I'm a normal, healthy person who happens to have some issues with food. I know I can address them through changing my behaviors," then go for it! You can do it!

Health Pyramid

Recite this sentence: *I am my most important priority.* As you say this, imagine yourself standing at the very top of a pyramid. This pyramid represents your health habits. Do you feel comfortable at the very top?

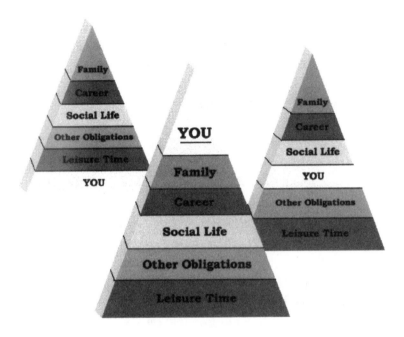

I put myself at the very top of my health pyramid eight years ago. I still socialize, volunteer my time, and run a successful business. But I'm always aware that my health is my number one priority. That's why I've been able to maintain a seventy-pound weight loss.

When a friend invites me to lunch, the first thing I do is assess my schedule. If I have too many places to go, too much going on, and an exercise opportunity is beginning to look impossible, I pass on the luncheon date. "Maybe next week," I promise my friend, "on a day when I won't feel so rushed." I never agree to a schedule that could jeopardize my health routine. Exercise and healthy eating come first and I make no compromises.

Seventy pounds ago, I was a totally different person.

Back then I never planned meals, healthy or otherwise, nor did I exercise. I lived moment to moment while focusing on my multiple jobs, shopping, college, my shoes, my car—*anything* but fitness and health. In terms of my health pyramid, I was buried somewhere beneath it. I felt too overwhelmed to make health my focus.

Everything and anything else came first.

If you're a "bottom-of-the-pyramid" dweller, you've probably *never* considered putting yourself at the very top of your pyramid. There *are* "middle-pyramid" dwellers who, when their schedules allow, *temporarily* make their health a priority, *temporarily* putting themselves at the top of their pyramid. The chronic dieter falls under this category. They may follow a healthy routine, committing for a limited time; they walk, join a gym, focus on good eating, but soon, they return to their old ways. They eventually demote themselves, returning to the middle of their pyramid, wondering how they wound up back there . . . again.

If you're a middle-pyramid dweller list all your daily activities. Next to each activity write: "more important than my health, yes or no"? If you're not prepared to make yourself more important than any of these activities, you may *not* be ready for weight loss.

You have the power to decide how you prioritize your time. Are you important enough to designate time in your schedule for exercise? Are you important enough to provide yourself with healthy meals? If that means you have to go to the store on a scheduled day, every week, are you prepared to make that commitment?

Where are *you* positioned on your priority pyramid?

It isn't just people with hectic schedules who place themselves low on their priority list. You may have little going on in your life. You may have shut down emotionally, with *nothing* qualifying as a priority. Being overweight can result in a depressed state of mind. You may feel that nothing matters, including you. But, like it or not, the same health rules still apply to you.

Make a list of the things in your life that compete for your time and attention. Don't worry about establishing a priority order as you list these things. Do that after you list them.

Now, put each thing you listed in order of importance. If *you* weren't on your list, put yourself there now. Where do you fit in?

Let's pretend that every time you answer to a commitment that *doesn't* make some contribution to your healthy weight-loss goal, a little piece of you is taken away. Move down your priority pyramid, until you reach your spot. How much of *you* is left? Is a big chunk of you missing? By the time you reach your name on that list, is there anything left of you at all? Other priorities can actually nibble your energy away, so that you have none left for pursuing fitness. Keeping yourself at the top ensures that you have the ability and strength to achieve fitness first. Being healthy and fit will actually give you the ability to meet other responsibilities more consistently and efficiently.

When I was at my peak weight, my social life ranked at the top of my pyramid. I went out with my friends three or more times a week. Many of my friendships were based on this "partying" pyramid structure, so for me to change things meant putting some of those friendships in jeopardy. We usually have to give up something to restructure our pyramid, and that can feel threatening. We may ask ourselves, *What will happen if I make that change?* The question we *should* ask ourselves is, *What will happen if I don't?*

Where would I be if I had been unwilling to risk change, if I had been unwilling to restructure my pyramid? I'd probably be even more overweight than I was at my peak. My friends would probably have moved on to other things, and I'd be in my thirties, still wishing I could change my life.

Did I lose some of my "partying" friends? Yes. After all, partying was all we really had in common. Basically, I sacrificed some bad habits in order to change my priorities.

What would *you* have to give up, or demote, to put yourself on top?

Close your eyes. Imagine yourself climbing to the top of a big, stone pyramid, passing all those things you currently put ahead of health and fitness. Imagine yourself standing firmly at the very top, feeling fit and energized. Imagine how much easier most of those other tasks are to deal with, now that you feel so healthy and good about yourself. What a feeling! What could be more important than this?

Adjust to the fact that you're worth it! When you *truly* believe you deserve to be everything you want to be, you can successfully use the information in this book to guide you toward a healthy, new life.

8

What to Expect after Weight Loss

Stage One

Believe it or not, the first year after my weight loss presented tough, new challenges. I suffered from a condition I'll call the "return to old behaviors phobia." If I received a dinner invitation, I'd panic. I'd call ahead to see what choices the restaurant offered. Unless the menu provided at least one healthy option, I wouldn't go. I *did* follow my own advice, always eating *before* going out. Still, how could I ignore my food history?

Ooh, they have my favorite. I do want to eat healthy, but I haven't had that food for so long! Temptation still frightened me. I was insecure.

I regularly tried to reassure myself, *Jen, things are different now.* But, I'd let myself down so many times in my "dieting" past. Could I trust this "new" me? Would I let myself down again?

True, I'd succeeded at losing weight, replaced many of my unhealthy behaviors with new healthy ones, but how deep did those changes go? Had I really changed? Was I fooling myself? Was I really a new person?

I was following all of my own weight-loss strategies. I was food shopping faithfully, buying healthy, nutritious choices. I was planning meals, and preparing them in advance, avoiding "starvation" mode. To keep my destructive behaviors under control, I ate a healthy, satisfying snack before attending social events. And, for the first time in my life, I had stayed committed to an exercise program for *an entire year!*

My body was where I wanted it to be, but my mind . . . ? It was in a constant state of turmoil. I felt like I was living with two very determined Jennifers, but they had conflicting goals. I regularly had to comfort and reassure myself. *Jennifer, you slipped and ate a bag of cookies, but it's okay. You don't have to be perfect. You've changed, remember . . . ?*

But, that part of me that expected perfection still struggled to control my behaviors. The newfound "accepting" part of me, the part that I was desperately trying to learn to live with, the part that was low pressure and kind, suggested I ignore the guilt/perfection side.

This conflict created a tremendous and unexpected internal struggle. I had spent most of my life wrestling with the idea that I had to be perfect or else and when I wasn't, I might as well give up. The "black or white" me had a motto: if you can't be perfect, you failed.

I knew approaching weight loss with that mind-set didn't work. My new, more positive approach had taken me to weight-loss success. But my negative voice wasn't going to surrender that easily. That unforgiving, perfection-focused part of me wasn't ready to be left behind.

For more than sixteen years I had listened to that negative voice. Sixteen years! Granted, for twenty-two months I had experienced a new life of structure, dedication, and determination. That new positive focus had taken me to the healthiest place I'd ever been. But the place I had come to was very new and unfamiliar. During those twenty-two months, I *had* succeeded in changing my body, but part of my mind had stubbornly refused to take the weight-loss journey with me. It was still standing somewhere in my past, waiting for that overweight Jennifer to return. That part of me expected failure, and now it was waiting for me to fail again. Because of that conflict I spent most of that "first year" in fear, second-guessing myself.

My former "eating buddies"? I avoided them. I also avoided my "partying" friends. I stayed home. I rented movies. I spent most of my free time alone. Some friends resented my new behavior. They called me the "President of the Weekend Loser Club." But I was hibernating because it made me feel safe. They could not understand; I was walking a tightrope. What if I couldn't maintain control? Any time an overweight person loses weight in any way, there will always be that fear. *Can I, will I keep it off?*

This weight loss *was* different. It was the result of behavior modification, not a diet. Why hadn't this new approach, this complete lifestyle change, solved all my internal conflicts? I was frightened. Instinctively, I understood that while strict routine had provided control, it hadn't really changed the way I related to food. That's where the fear came from.

And sometimes, after that successful weight loss, I *did* lose control; I'd eat an entire carton of ice cream in one sitting, or half a jar of peanut butter with chocolate chips mixed in. The thing that terrified me most was that my good behaviors weren't consistent. I could suddenly lapse into destructive eating behaviors at any time. When I did, I was more than willing to listen to that old, negative voice scream, *Jennifer, you self-sabotaging idiot!*

After any out-of-control food episode, I became frightened. Who was I kidding? I hadn't changed! How could I stay faithful to healthy eating behaviors for a lifetime? Impossible! I hadn't even been able to keep regular dieting promises for a short time! Granted I hadn't *raced* to my weight goal; it had been a slow walk into a new world. But, did I belong here?

I began to realize that I was focusing on the negative. Had I forgotten, during the twenty-two months it had taken me to lose weight, I had made a *promise* to myself to "let go of the perfect"? I had to remind myself to listen to my friendlier, more forgiving voice. Occasional overeating episodes were to be expected. *Accept the fact that you will occasionally let yourself down,* I told myself. *Just make sure these behaviors don't continue for days, weeks, or months. Your weight loss will survive an occasional lapse, but it won't survive 'giving up' and returning to old behaviors on a regular basis.*

In spite of what I had come to believe, at Stage One I was still often asking myself, *Can I maintain this weight loss?*

Stage Two

I made it through that first year without returning to my old ways. How? I didn't let the occasional "F-grade" food day allow me to quit.

When I ate ten cookies, I brushed myself off and moved forward. I had worked too hard to give up that easily. I had invested a lot of time and energy in myself. Now I was prepared to accept the fact that getting used to new behaviors was going to take time. I had been "out of control" for more than sixteen years. Also, I had to accept the fact that I would continue to make mistakes. Gradually, very gradually, I was letting go of the concept of "perfect."

Here is another important point I have to make. For the first time, I was developing a sense of humor. I'm not going to claim I suddenly found the imperfections in my eating habits amusing, but for the first time, anger with myself wasn't my first response. Why declare myself an "irresponsible food freak" just because I'd eaten five slices of pizza? What good would *that* do? Maybe overeating wasn't the crime of the century after all. Granted I was, and still am, frustrated by my bad food behaviors, but the frustration no longer evolves into anger and self-loathing. I've learned to let go of my disappointment, before it becomes more destructive. Do I still *want* to be perfect? Yes. Do I *still* believe that perfection (in my behaviors or my body) is a realistic and/or healthy goal? *No!*

Two years later, I had achieved a certain level of credibility. "Jennifer," a friend would tell me, "this restaurant has healthy stuff, you'll like this place!" When I socialized, friends no longer asked why I ordered soda water. It was expected. Friends now understood why I took my own car when we went out. If they planned to stop for greasy food at the end of the evening, I wanted the option of going home to avoid temptation. They no longer asked why I brought my own veggie burgers and low-fat potato salad to a cookout. They no longer said, "Ah, come on!" when I said, "I'll meet you guys *after* I go to the gym." I got used to the compliments I received. I enjoyed the validation and the endorsing feedback. But I knew the most important thing was keeping in touch with that new, more positive *me*. That "me" had put Jennifer, her health and her habits, at the very top of her priority pyramid.

Friends and family now expected certain behaviors from me, which, in turn, had its own positive effect. I started to expect certain behaviors of *myself*. Because I had more confidence, people weren't doubting me. Because people weren't doubting me, I was doubting myself less often. My new healthy behaviors began to feel natural. Slowly, they were becoming a way of life. Although I *still* earned the occasional "F" on a destructive food day, that grade didn't scare me so much anymore. So, at Stage Two, I was beginning to trust myself. *Maybe I can maintain this weight for life.*

Eight Years Later

I've maintained the same size for more than eight years. Today, being healthy and fit feels natural.

I display photographs in my office, of the "old" me. They remind me how hard I worked, and how far I've come. The photos also serve as an inspiration for clients. "Was that *you*, Jennifer?"

In one photo, the one on the cover of this book, I was on vacation in Holland and weighed over 200 pounds. I was at my heaviest. Clients are often shocked when they see this picture. "You looked so old! I can't believe that was you! Other than the smile, you look nothing like the woman in that picture!"

When I first lost weight, I carried that photograph everywhere. When I lectured on weight loss, I introduced myself by holding up an enlargement of that "peak-weight" photo. I enjoyed the gasps from the audience, and the wide-eyed stares the picture produced. It made me feel proud of myself.

Today, eight years later, I look at that photo differently. Years ago, introducing myself while holding that photo, served as a reminder: *Jennifer, this was you. You must NEVER look like this again.* I no longer need that reminder.

I've become set in my healthy ways; I no longer identify with that large and frustrated young woman in the photo. But, eight years later, food issues are still with me.

I assumed that in time I'd have a "normal" relationship with food. I expected to be able to eat just like my mom. I'd be one of "those" people, the ones who eat just half of a cookie, not wanting more, because they feel "full." I thought I'd be the person who leaves the last two bites of food on her plate, because she's had "just enough." I'd be able to eat foods like pizza without guilt. Food would be just . . . food. No more eating "out of control," no emotional attachment, no self-destructive behaviors.

That hasn't happened.

I hoped to become a person who could visit a gym with confidence. *Boy, I sure look great in Spandex! I'm so fit! I wish I could live in this fabric! Check me out everybody! They call me "hot bod!"* Boy it's sure crowded in here, but that doesn't matter—*I* love *large crowds of "beautiful" people.*

That hasn't happened.

There was a time when I assumed I'd eventually look back in disgust, unable to relate to the bad food behaviors of an overeater. I'd tell myself, *Gee, Jennifer, you sure had some tough times around food. Glad those days are over forever.*

Today while the overweight photo of me is hard to relate to, the relationship I had with food is not. I'm still that person. I still eat when I'm not hungry. I still finish what's on my plate. I still eat too quickly. I still find it hard to stop eating when I *really* like the taste. But my healthy routines have saved me. They make it possible for me to maintain a healthy balance. Without those routines, I wouldn't be where I am today.

It is important for you to understand that although I've maintained my weight loss for over eight years, I have not developed the mindset of a naturally thin person. My hunger meter is still broken. What has changed is the distribution of power. Today, I have power over my food choices. I no longer let food control me.

That food-threatened person we want desperately to get away from will always be part of us. If you expect weight loss to help you lose that person, the one who's let you down in the past, then weight loss will disappoint you. *That person will be a part of you for life. It's not about losing that person, it's about learning to live with, and developing a peaceful coexistence with that person.*

Will you let an occasional relapse into bad food behaviors "make" or "break" your weight loss? Will you quit, or will you stay on track and learn from your mistakes?

I could claim this is the "miracle book." I could tell you that, once you read this book and follow my advice, you're guaranteed permanent and easy weight-loss success, and you'll never have to worry about letting yourself down again.

Hallelujah! You've found the cure! But, here's the reality: food issues do *not* go away.

Can you accept that?

It's more about the "inside" you than the "outside" you. It's about you taking responsibility for your weight and working to change your life. It's about *you* being *your own* biggest supporter.

No more setting time limits. It's not about time. It's about other things, like learning to make movement a part of your life, reading food labels, going to the grocery store, preplanning your food, and never saying, "I'm on a diet." It all comes down to making yourself your number one priority.

Change your life and your body will thank you. Play games with your body, and your body will get even.

You can continue to search for that miracle—the one diet that will do it all *for* you.

If you still believe the cure is out there, you're not ready to lose weight. I can say this with 100 percent confidence: you're just not ready.

It took me nearly twenty years to figure that out. My awareness developed from my own personal weight-loss experiences, and through seven years of one-on-one counseling and sharing the experiences of clients. I have clients who are just as embarrassed as I was when they admit having tried every diet under the sun.

This is what you need to know: You're not alone. All of us who struggle with weight share the same experiences. We've all experienced failure and have questioned whether starting again was worth it.

The only thing that separates us from the people who have the body they want is our longing for perfection. It clouds the way we *perceive* our weight problem and the guilt and pain that accompanies that perception. I guarantee you've been much more rigid about food, in your "dieting life" than *any* naturally lean person has *ever* been. You've failed to achieve permanent weight loss, not because you haven't been hard enough on yourself, but because you've been too hard on yourself.

Believe in yourself, be kinder to yourself, and reward yourself with a life change. If I can succeed, so can you.

Self-help Questions

Test Yourself

I always start new client relationships with a question-and-answer session. The following includes some questions that are designed to help you get in touch with your behaviors. They will help you identify common, damaging patterns that produce weight gain. Record your answers. Be absolutely honest. Make no judgments. Do not think in terms of *right* or *wrong*. If you need to, refer to the chapter to which the question relates.

Chapter 1: Why We're Different

(See pages 1–14.)

1. How do you feel when you envision yourself at your "ideal body" goal?

2. If you identify with the broken hunger meter, how do you think it affects your eating habits?

3. Can you create a list of non-hunger eating episodes?

4. Describe the eating habits of a naturally lean person. Do you believe that you or they are more likely to demand "perfect" food behaviors?

5. Is fear of not getting enough an issue for you? If it is, when do you think this fear began?

Chapter 2: Desperate for Control

(See pages 15–46.)

1. Are you prepared to begin your new, healthy lifestyle? If you are prepared to begin, set a date you're comfortable with.

2. Can you let go of weight-loss time limits? If you can't, what's your fear? Write it down, without making any judgments about it.

3. How many diets have you tried? How did they make you feel—at the beginning of the diet and at the end? Did you truly believe that a diet would permanently solve your weight problem?

4. Do you demand perfection from yourself while you're dieting? Do you agree that striving for perfection can sabotage you? How?

5. Can you recall an out-of-control food experience? Imagine yourself back in that situation. What could you have done to change the outcome?

6. Have you had success (long-term) on *any* weight-loss program? What qualified it as successful or unsuccessful?

7. Take a picture of yourself and record your measurements. Avoid use of your scale for at least a month. Focus on your measurements instead. Measure yourself monthly and record your progress.

8. Purchase a small amount of a favorite food, one that has often caused you to lose control. *Slowly* and *thoughtfully* eat that small portion of your out-of-control food. Think about the eating experience as you are having it. How does the food taste? What do you enjoy most about that food? How does it make you feel? How do you feel *after* you eat it? Record your feelings.

Chapter 3: New Habits, New Body

(See pages 47–84.)

1. Guess—without actually checking—how many calories you typically consume in a day. Then determine how accurate your guess was by reading labels and other product information.

2. Create a lower calorie, lower fat version of your favorite meal.

3. Promise you will never let yourself reach starvation mode. Focus on eating nutritious foods at two- to three-hour intervals.

4. How would you describe your "fireplace"?

5. If you have a fireplace #1, how will you begin to change it?

6. Make a list of your I-can't-stop foods. Can you make a commitment to keep those foods out of reach until you learn to be more in control around them?

Chapter 4: The Safety of Routine

(See pages 85–94.)

1. Pick a grocery store day. Explain why that day is a good one. Pick a backup day. Why is your backup day likely to work?

2. Pick a food-prep day. (This is a day, once every week, that provides fifteen to twenty minutes for washing, slicing and dicing, so you can create healthy food choices.) Mark it on your calendar.

3. Think about tomorrow's schedule before going to bed. Design a healthy food plan that will fit within that schedule. For example, if you have to chauffeur kids, go to a meeting, watch a two-hour soccer game or run errands, be sure to pack healthy snacks and take them with you. That will allow you to stay ahead of your hunger.

Chapter 5: Nobody's Business

(See pages 95–100.)

1. Who will support you during a life change? If you feel safe and comfortable doing it, tell them, and only them, what you plan to do. Otherwise, keep your health goals to yourself. Weight loss is not a public issue.

2. Write an outrageous, ridiculous excuse for not eating fattening foods at a party. Be creative.

Chapter 6: You Gotta Get Moving!

(See pages 101–116.)

1. Do you hate exercise? If you do, list the reasons. Examine your list and circle the reasons that can be eliminated.

2. What calorie burning activities do you enjoy? Can you see yourself engaging in that activity for five minutes, four to five times a week? Can you imagine yourself slowly increasing your time commitment to that activity?

3. How many times have you attempted to lose weight? How many of those attempts have included a commitment to exercise?

4. How many minutes, and how many days a week, are you willing to allot to an exercise routine? Write your answer. How do you feel about what you've written? Is your answer realistic? What kind of exercise promises have you made to yourself in the past? What happened?

5. Set a *realistic* goal contract with yourself: I _____ will exercise _____ times a week for _____ minutes. I accept the fact that, no matter how minimal and modest my goal seems, it still represents a wonderful new beginning.

Chapter 7: Where's Your Head?

(See pages 117–127.)

1. Why do you think you are overweight? Can you live with that explanation? Does your answer make it more difficult or less difficult for you to achieve weight loss?

2. Where have you put yourself on your priority pyramid?

3. What fear has been your greatest barrier to maintained weight loss?

4. Are you generally very hard on yourself when you make a mistake? Using a "kind voice," write a sentence that offers a solution to a mistake you've made.

5. Does the thought of weight loss make you feel overwhelmed? If so, how has that feeling impacted your dieting history?

Chapter 8: What to Expect after Weight Loss

(See pages 129–135.)

1. Did my confession that I still have food issues—even after reaching and maintaining weight loss—surprise you? Describe how that information makes you feel.

2. On a scale of one to ten, rank weight loss in terms of importance in your life (number one being of highest importance). Explain why you have given it that rating.

3. On the same scale, rank your level of determination. Explain why you have given it that rating.

4. Rank what you sincerely believe to be your likelihood of success. Why have you given it that rating?

5. Where do you see yourself five years from now if you *don't* successfully address your weight problem?

6. Where do you see yourself five years from now if you *do* successfully address your weight problem?

7. Write a brief description of yourself (your personality *and* your body) using only positive terms.

8. How do you feel about the information you've been given?

9. Do you believe you *can* lose weight and maintain that weight loss for life with a new, realistic approach?

10. How do you feel about yourself and your life in general?

Have faith in yourself. You can do it. You *can* change your life.

About the Author

Having successfully lost more than seventy pounds, Jennifer Klein was chosen to participate in a weight-control behavioral study at the University of Pittsburgh Medical Center.[*]

For more than seven years she has professionally coached weight loss, one on one. Through her business, Gain Control Not Weight, she has given hundreds of clients the confidence and skills needed to lose weight and become fit. She is a certified personal trainer and a certified nutrition specialist. She is a graduate of the University of Massachusetts—Boston with a degree in English and women's studies.

In 1995 she was featured as a Success Story in *Shape* magazine. Her weight-loss accomplishment was also profiled in *First* magazine in 1998. She was twice invited to appear on NBC's *Real Life* and has produced and hosted her own local television program. As a lecturer, she has addressed weight-loss topics at health clubs and major corporations. Boston's News Center 7 lists Jennifer Klein as one of its weight-loss information resources.

She lives in the Boston area with her husband.

[*] Additional information about this study may be found by calling the University of Pittsburgh at 1-800-606-NWCR.